European School of Oncology

Monographs

Series Editor: U. Veronesi

The European School of Oncology gratefully acknowledges sponsorship for the Task Force received from

ICI Pharmaceuticals

A. Goldhirsch (Ed.)

Endocrine Therapy of Breast Cancer V

With 33 Figures and 20 Tables

Springer-Verlag
Berlin Heidelberg New York
London Paris Tokyo
Hong Kong Barcelona
Budapest

A. Goldhirsch

Department of Medical Oncology
Ospedale Civico
via Tesserete 46
6900 Lugano, Switzerland

ISBN 3-540-55718-0 Springer-Verlag Berlin Heidelberg New York
ISBN 0-387-55718-0 Springer-Verlag New York Berlin Heidelberg

Typesetting: Camera ready by editor
Printing: Druckhaus Beltz, Hemsbach/Bergstr.; Binding: J. Schäffer GmbH & Co. KG, Grünstadt
23/3145-5 4 3 2 1 0 – Printed on acid-free paper

Foreword

The European School of Oncology came into existence to respond to a need for information, education and training in the field of the diagnosis and treatment of cancer. There are two main reasons why such an initiative was considered necessary. Firstly, the teaching of oncology requires a rigorously multidisciplinary approach which is difficult for the Universities to put into practice since their system is mainly disciplinary orientated. Secondly, the rate of technological development that impinges on the diagnosis and treatment of cancer has been so rapid that it is not an easy task for medical faculties to adapt their curricula flexibly.

With its residential courses for organ pathologies and the seminars on new techniques (laser, monoclonal antibodies, imaging techniques etc.) or on the principal therapeutic controversies (conservative or mutilating surgery, primary or adjuvant chemotherapy, radiotherapy alone or integrated), it is the ambition of the European School of Oncology to fill a cultural and scientific gap and, thereby, create a bridge between the University and Industry and between these two and daily medical practice.

One of the more recent initiatives of ESO has been the institution of permanent study groups, also called task forces, where a limited number of leading experts are invited to meet once a year with the aim of defining the state of the art and possibly reaching a consensus on future developments in specific fields of oncology.

The ESO Monograph series was designed with the specific purpose of disseminating the results of these study group meetings, and providing concise and updated reviews of the topic discussed.

It was decided to keep the layout relatively simple, in order to restrict the costs and make the monographs available in the shortest possible time, thus overcoming a common problem in medical literature: that of the material being outdated even before publication.

UMBERTO VERONESI
Chairman Scientific Committee
European School of Oncology

Contents

Introduction

A. Goldhirsch

Division of Oncology, Ospedale San Giovanni, Bellinzona, Ospedale Regionale, Lugano, and Ospedale Regionale Beata Vergine, Mendrisio, Switzerland

This is the fifth issue of our Monograph on Endocrine Therapy of Breast Cancer. It presents reports that stimulated many interesting discussions among the Task Force members and some guests who met in Orta, Italy, in early 1991 under the auspices of the European School of Oncology. Once again, the meeting resulted in a very exciting and pleasant intellectual exercise during which a variety of levels of current knowledge and future research were thoroughly discussed. The spectrum of the items on the agenda was remarkably broad and included the normal breast cell, the cancer cell, mechanisms of resistance to therapeutic agents, new treatments, the patient with breast cancer, her quality of life, and some public health issues related to the population of women with the disease. The Monograph provides summaries of some of the discussed topics and reflects the stimulating atmosphere during the Task Force meeting.

Dr. Taylor-Papadimitriou discusses normal cell lineages and the phenotype of the breast cancer cell with its peculiar products. Dr. Milgrom writes about the breast cancer oestrogen-induced protein, pB2, its identification and putative role. Dr. Jordan covers two topics related to the mechanisms by which endocrine agents may exert their effect in a premalignant stage and during adjuvant therapies. Dr. Kaye treats the interesting issue of multidrug resistance and especially its reversal by various agents including antioestrogens. Dr. Manni provides an update on new endocrine agents, pointing out some very interesting candidates. Dr. Rose evaluates prognostic factors in early breast cancer. Drs. Howell and Schor discuss the clinical relevance of epithelial-stromal interrelationships and reciprocal stimuli and suppressions. Drs. Gelber, Castiglione and Goldhirsch argue, as in previous editions of the Monograph, in favour of a meaningful reporting of results from trials of adjuvant therapies in breast cancer, putting increasing emphasis on quality of life. They also discuss the emerging superiority of combined chemo-endocrine therapies in terms of treatment effects.

The field of breast cancer in general and endocrine mechanisms in particular continues to represent a most interesting and fertile ground for the implementation of knowledge on human malignant diseases. All authors hope that this Monograph will be as useful for such purpose to the readership as the discussions within the Task Force were for the participants.

Normal Cell Lineages and the Phenotype of the Breast Cancer Cell

Joyce Taylor-Papadimitriou

Imperial Cancer Research Fund, P.O. Box 123, 44 Lincoln's Inn Fields, London WC2A 3PX, United Kingdom

The importance of defining the malignant phenotype within the framework of the lineages of the normal cell from which it derives has been clearly demonstrated in the haemopoietic system where the subclassification of leukaemias achieved in this way has led to a more objective approach to disease management and therapy. The success of the approach has depended on 3 major factors, namely, 1) the availability of specific immunological markers (monoclonal antibodies) to define differentiation-related antigens, 2) the easy availability of circulating blood cells and 3) the development of culture systems where primitive and more differentiated progenitor cells could be cultured and induced to clonally differentiate.

Progress in applying a similar approach to the study of epithelial cancers has been slow. However, the development of monoclonal antibodies to epithelial antigens means that the tools are beginning to be available to subclassify cells in the tissues. In the case of the mammary gland it is also relatively easy to obtain tissue from non-malignant breast as well as from breast cancers. The problems which remain relate to: 1) the complexity of the tissue of the mammary gland and the interaction between the different components and 2) the fact that development of the gland is restricted to certain periods such as puberty, pregnancy and lactation, which are difficult to reproduce *in vitro*. At the moment therefore, while subclasses of cells can be defined by monoclonal antibodies in tissue sections of normal breast tissue, the dynamic relationship between these subclasses (at least in the human) is difficult to establish.

In spite of the above limitations, it is still possible to characterise breast cancers using antibodies which recognise antigens expressed by specific subclasses of the normal epithelial cells lining the mammary tree. In this way subclassifications of breast cancers are becoming possible based on antigen expression, and in some cases the subclassification relates to prognosis. By inference the results of these studies on the cancers can be used in helping to formulate, in a speculative manner, the possible cell lineages in the normal gland. In this chapter, I will review the results of staining normal and malignant breast tissue with antibodies to certain antigens expressed by normal mammary epithelial cells and attempt to integrate the data into a framework suggesting possible relationships between different epithelial subsets. The culture systems available and problems associated with them will also be briefly discussed.

Epithelial Cell Types in the Human Mammary Gland

Two major classes of epithelial cells have been recognised in the mammary gland on the basis of their position and function, namely the basal or myoepithelial cells and the luminal or secretory epithelial cell. As will be seen, immunohistochemical staining confirms this classification by demonstrating major differences in antigen expression in the basal and luminal epithelial cells.

The antigens expressed by the normal epithelial cells which are to be discussed in detail are listed in Table 1. This is by no means an exhaustive list, but represents those antigens which have also been studied reason-

Table 1. Breast cancer-associated antigens which are also expressed by normal breast epithelial cells

Antigen	Expressed on basal epithelium	luminal epithelium	% cancers expressing the antigen
POLYMORPHIC EPITHELIAL MUCIN (PEM)	-	+	>90%
OESTROGEN RECEPTOR	-	+ (≈6%)	>50%
INTERMEDIATE FILAMENTS			
Keratins 7,8,18,19	- [a]	+ [b]	>90%
Keratins 5,14	+	- [c]	≈10%
Vimentin	+	-	≈10%
EGF RECEPTOR	++	+	20-30%

a Some keratin 19 expression is seen in the basal cells of the large ducts.

b Keratins 8 and 18 are expressed homogeneously. Keratin 19 is expressed homogeneously in the luminal cells of the large ducts, but in the terminal ductal lobular units, some keratin 19 negative cells are seen.

c Some keratin 14 expression is seen in the luminal cells of the large ducts.

ably intensively in breast tumours and which may define a subset of cells in the normal breast. Of the antigens listed in Table 1, the mucin PEM, keratins 8, 18 and 19 and the oestrogen receptor (ER) are found only in luminal epithelial cells although weak expression of keratin 19 can be seen in the basal cells of the large ducts. The expression of keratins 5 and 14 and vimentin, on the other hand, is mainly restricted to the basal cells which also express a higher level of epidermal growth factor receptors (EGF-R) than do the luminal cells.

Expression of PEM by Normal and Malignant Breast Epithelial Cells

Attention has been focussed on the human epithelial mucins because they are highly immunogenic in the mouse and many antibodies are available which react with them. Mucins are characterised by a high content of carbohydrate which is attached, in O-linkage, to a core protein. The dominant mucin expressed by mammary epithelial cells is a highly polymorphic mucin which we have called PEM [1,2]. We and others have cloned and sequenced the gene coding for the core protein of the mammary mucin [3-7] and the gene has been called MUC1 [8] although we still refer to the product of the gene in the mammary gland as PEM. Sequence analysis shows that PEM is a transmembrane protein with a short cytoplasmic tail and with a large part of the extracellular domain being made up of tandem repeats. Since each repeat contains O-glycosylation sites, it is this domain which is heavily glycosylated.

In the normal gland, PEM is expressed on the luminal aspect of the luminal cells, and although it is expressed in the resting breast, it is dramatically upregulated at pregnancy and lactation. In fact the best source of PEM is either milk or the milk fat globule found in the cream fraction of milk. An examination of a large number of tumours shows that more than 90% express PEM suggesting that these tumours may have developed from luminal cells [9].

There are two interesting features about PEM expression in breast cancers. Firstly, the expression is generally much higher than seen in the normal resting breast, and secondly the cancer-associated mucin appears to be aberrantly glycosylated. The high level of expression seen in cancers could indicate that the majority of cells in the tumour which show high positive staining may represent a more differentiated phenotype than the luminal cells seen in the resting breast. This explanation would be supported by the results of staining with antibodies to keratin 19 (see below). The second point of interest, the aberrant glycosylation of the mucin, has important practical implications. Analysis of the carbohydrate side chains on the normal and cancer-associated mucin shows that the side chains of the cancer-associated mucin are shorter [10,11]. This means that the tumour mucin is antigenically dissimilar to the normal mucin and antibodies are available which can show selectivity in their reaction with the tumour mucin. These may react with novel epitopes which are found in the carbohydrate side chains, or with epitopes in the core protein which are unmasked because of the early termination of the carbohydrate side chains [12]. The tumour mucin also appears to contain T cell epitopes which are recognised by T cell lines isolated from breast cancer patients [13]. These features of the cancer associated mucin make it an important target for antibodies and these have been used effectively to image ovarian cancers which also express the aberrantly glycosylated mucin [14]. Studies are also underway to evaluate the possible use of PEM or antigens based on its structure in active specific immunotherapy of breast and ovarian tumours.

The relevance of the studies on PEM to the main theme of this review is that its expression by breast cancers suggests that the cancers expressing the mucin develop from the luminal cells. There is also evidence that the expression of extracellular mucin carrying an epitope found on the normally processed mucin defines a subset of cancers with improved prognosis [15].

Intermediate Filaments

The Family of Intermediate Filaments

The various classes of intermediate filament proteins (IFPs) are listed in Table 2. They show considerable structural similarity but are antigenically distinguishable, so that monoclonal antibodies can be developed which exclusively recognise a single species.

Initial studies on the expression of IFPs by different cell types, suggested that the class of intermediate filament expressed were (with a few exceptions) specific for a particular cell or

Table 2. Intermediate filament types

Gene family	Filament proteins	Tissue type
Type I	Keratins: small acidic	Epithelia
Type II	Keratins: Neutral to basic	Epithelia
Type III	Vimentin	Mesenchyme
	Desmin	Muscle
	Glial filament protein	Astroglia
	Peripherin	CNS stem cells
Type IV	Neurofilament proteins	Neurons
Type V	A and B type laminins	Most cells
Type VI	Nestin	CNS stem cells

tissue type as illustrated in Table 2 [16]. It also seemed that this tissue specificity was maintained in the change to malignancy, even when other parameters of differentiation were lost, making the IFPs extremely important antigens in tumour diagnosis. While both of these assumptions have proved to be generally valid, there are now examples where representatives of more than one class of IFP have been found to be expressed in the same cell or tissue. These findings make it necessary to exercise caution in interpreting IFP expression to define differentiated and malignant phenotypes. Providing such caution is exercised, however, antibodies which are reactive with IFPs provide useful tools for approaching the difficult problem of cell characterisation.

Keratin Expression in Epithelial Tissues

The cytokeratins, which form the intermediate filaments (tonofilaments) of epithelial cells, represent the most complex family of IFPs. In human epithelia, 20 soft tissue keratins have been identified and classified [17,18]. On the basis of their molecular weight and isoelectric point determined by gel electrophoresis, the human keratins have been given the numbers 1-20. Numbers 1-8 form the keratin type II group of larger basic keratins, while numbers 9-20 form the keratin type I group of smaller acidic keratins. In contrast to other IFP types, keratins must form heteropolymers of at least one keratin from each group to form a filament. As a result, epithelial cells express at least 2 different (and in most cases more than 2) keratin polypeptides.
In Figure 1 the basic features of keratin expression in 3 different kinds of epithelia, are illustrated. Two generalisations can be made, namely, that all simple epithelia express keratins 8 and 18 and all basal cells, whether in a stratified or "mixed" epithelium (like the mammary gland) express keratins 5 and 14. Keratins 7 and 19 may also be expressed in some simple epithelia, and heterogeneous expression of keratin 19 can also be found in basal cells of some stratified epithelia. In stratifying epithelia different pairs of keratins are expressed depending on the tissue.

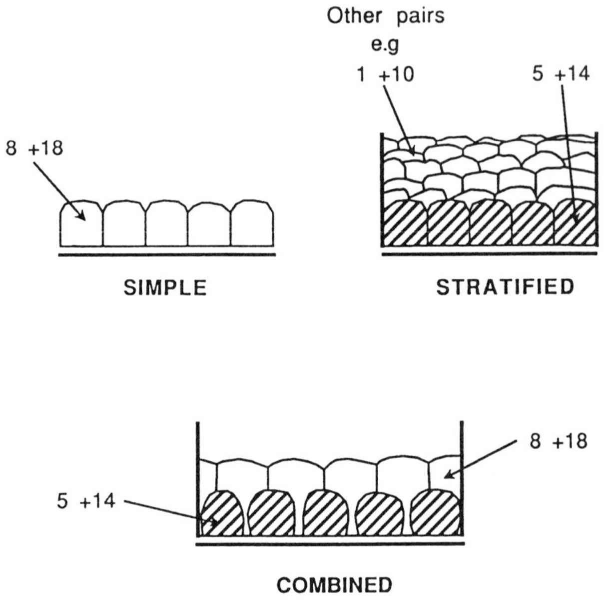

Fig. 1. Expression of keratins in different types of epithelial cells

Intermediate Filament Expression in the Mammary Gland

Distinction between basal and luminal cells

The mammary gland, like the salivary or sweat gland, is a mixed epithelium (see Fig. 1). The basal cells sit directly on the basement membrane, and express keratin 5 and 14; recently they have also been shown to express vimentin [19]. The luminal cells which rest on the basal cells, and have processes which extend to the basement membrane, have a free luminal surface and express keratins 7, 8, 18 and 19. In the terminal ductal lobular units (TDLU), most luminal cells do not express keratins 5 and 14 and vimentin, and basal cells do not express keratins 7, 8, 18 and 19 so that there is a difference in the profile of intermediate filament expression by the 2 major cell types. However, subsets in both luminal and basal cells have been identified. Also, in the larger ducts the distinction is less clear, the basal cells show weak expression of keratin 19, while luminal cells show weak expression of keratin 14 [20].

Subsets of epithelial cells defined by IF expression

Although the expression of vimentin does appear to be restricted to the basal cells, there is some disagreement as to whether all the basal cells express this protein. It is not clear, therefore, whether vimentin expression characterises a subset of basal cells or not. Gould and colleagues [21], however, have recently found that a subset of basal cells in the TDLU express glial filament protein (GFP).
In the luminal cells of the TDLU, one subset of cells has been defined by their ability to express keratin 5 [21,22] and another by their lack of ability to express keratin 19 [23]. The keratin 19-negative luminal cells are particularly interesting, since this cell type appears at puberty when ductal branching occurs [24], and has a high proliferative capacity *in vitro* [23]. A diagram showing the expression of IFP in the resting human mammary gland is shown in Figure 2. Figures 3a and b also illustrate the expression of keratins 14 and 19 in the resting gland.

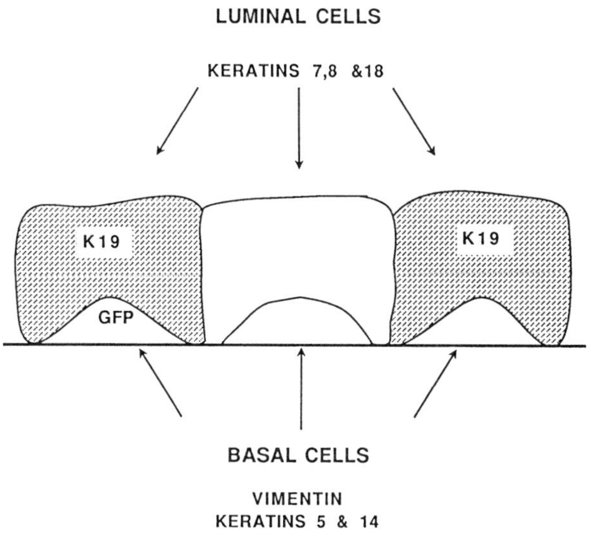

Fig. 2. Expression of intermediate filaments in the basal and luminal cells of the normal adult human mammary gland

IFP expression by tumours

The expression of individual keratins in breast cancers has been examined in a large number of tumours using monoclonal antibodies monospecific for a single keratin species. The results show that the majority of breast cancers (around 90%) express the simple epithelial keratins 8, 18 and 19 (and sometimes 7) expressed by the normal luminal cells, and do not express the basal epithelial keratin 14 or vimentin [20] (see Figs. 3e and f): keratin 5 has not been examined in a large number of tumours. Thus, most of the cancers express a profile of intermediate filaments, characteristic of the normal luminal epithelial cell seen in the TDLU. As might be expected, benign tumours which maintain elements of structure express basal keratins where basal cells are present (see Fig. 3c).
The expression of keratin 19 by the majority of tumours [25,26] is rather surprising since the keratin 19-positive cells appear to be more differentiated than the keratin 19-negative cells which in fact do not express casein at lactation or secretory component in the resting breast [24]. It is interesting to note that benign tumours contain an increased number of keratin 19-negative luminal cells probably reflecting their polyclonal origin and the high proliferative potential of the keratin 19 negative cells. The expression of keratin 19 and the upregulation of expression of PEM strongly suggests that most of the cells in invasive breast cancers show the phenotype of the differentiated luminal epithelial cell. The correlation of expression of keratin 19 with prognosis has not been studied.

Prognosis and IF expression

Although the majority of breast cancers have been found to show an intermediate filament profile chracteristic of luminal epithelial cells, a small subset have recently been identified which express vimentin [27-33] or keratin 14 [34,35]. Of great interest is the observation that the expression of these intermediate filament proteins characteristic of basal cells in the normal gland appears to be associated with poor prognosis [31,33,36]. Vimentin was not expressed in lobular carcinomas but rather associated with high-grade infiltrating ductal carcinomas [30]. Moreover, vimentin appears to be expressed in cancers with a low ER content, and a high K167-defined growth fraction and EGF-R content [29,31,32].

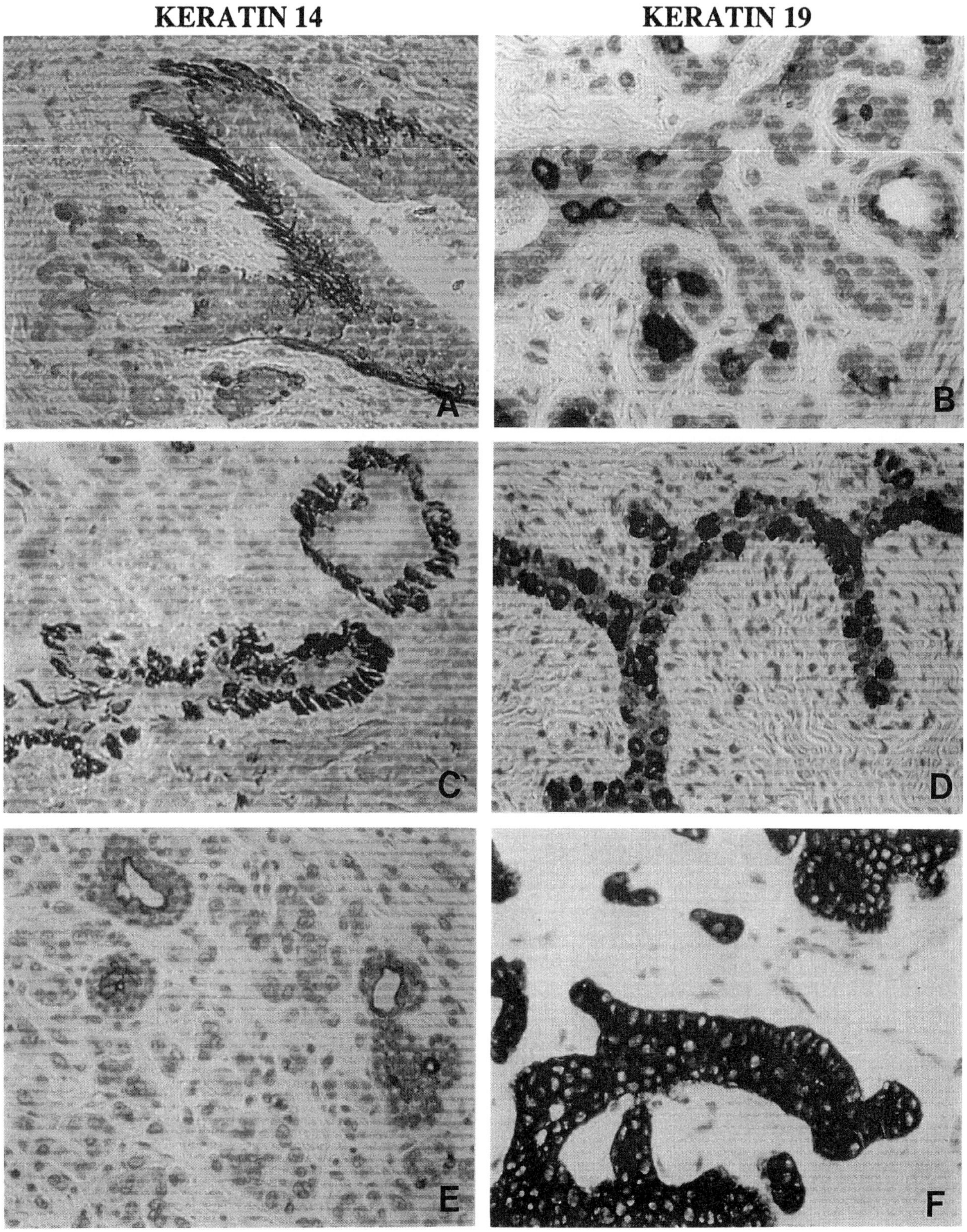

Fig. 3. Expression of keratin 14 (A,C,E) and keratin 19 (B,D,F) in the normal mammary gland (A,B), a fibroadenoma (C,D) and invasive ductal carcinoma (E,F)

Expression of Growth Factor Receptors in Normal and Malignant Mammary Epithelium

Several growth factors have been found to affect the proliferation of human mammary epithelial cells in culture. With the advent of monoclonal antibodies detecting growth factor receptors, it has been possible to analyse the expression of these on the normal epithelial cells. The two considered here, the oestrogen receptor (ER) and the EGF receptor (EGF-R), are expressed in some tumours and are widely used as prognostic indicators. C-erb-B2, which is related to EGF-R and also expressed on tumours showing a poor prognosis [37], is not discussed because it has not been detected on normal mammary epithelial cells. It is, however, interesting to note that antibodies to erb-B2 have identified a subset of *in situ* tumours which all stain strongly [38], as do all cases of mammary Paget's disease [39], suggesting that erb-B2 expression may be a feature of a subset of normal mammary epithelial cells (from which these tumours develop) which is hitherto unidentified.

Oestrogen Receptors

Although 50% of breast cancers are found to express the oestrogen receptor, only a very small fraction of cells in the normal resting, pre-menopausal breast (around 6-7%) have been found to show positive staining with antibodies to ER [40,41] and this is reduced dramatically at pregnancy and lactation [42]. There is some suggestion, however, that the percentage of ER+ cells increases post-menopausally (40). This would correlate with the higher percentage of ER-positive tumours found in post menopausal patients (60%) as compared to pre-menopausal patients (30%). The reason why such a high proportion of cancers express ER is not clear. The main point to emphasise for the purposes of this discussion is that ER+ cells are found in the luminal position in the normal breast. Since ER-positive tumours are generally found to show a better prognosis than ER-negative tumours, (and tend not to show evidence of expression of basal markers such as EGF-R (see below) and vimentin), these observations suggest that retention of expression of some luminal features by breast cancers is associated with a good prognosis.

Epidermal Growth Factor Receptor

Studies on the expression of the epidermal growth factor receptor in breast cancers have identified a subset of tumours which show a high expression of EGF-R [43-45]. The expression of EGF-R appears to be inversely related to ER expression [44-46] and is correlated with vimentin expression [29] and with a poor prognosis [46,47]. Studies following the distribution of EGF-R on normal mammary epithelial cells are somewhat limited, however, Isutsumi and colleagues [48] and Nicholson (personal communication) have found staining with an antibody to EGF-R to be stronger on myoepithelial than on luminal cells, (although both cell types show positive staining). It is possible, therefore, that the high expression of EGF-R in a subset of breast cancers reflects the expression of antigens characteristic of basal epithelial cells in these tumours, particularly since increased EGF-R expression is correlated with vimentin expression (another basal marker).

Whether the high expression of EGF-R in the tumour reflects a higher mitogenic response to the growth factor or merely acts as a marker for a less differentiated cell is not clear. Certainly EGF is a potent mitogen for normal and benign human mammary epithelial cells in culture [49,50] and both EGF and TGF-alpha (which binds to EGF-R) appear to play a role in mammary morphogenesis [51]. Although expression of EGF-R and ER are inversely related in breast cancers, over-expression of EGF-R in ER+ human breast cancer cell line does not induce an oestrogen-independent phenotype [52], suggesting that signals generated by EGF-R cannot replace the signals induced by ER in these cells.

Table 3 summarises somewhat simplistically the data discussed so far, suggesting that expression of markers associated with the basal cell phenotype in breast cancers appears to be associated with a poor prognosis. Such tumours, however, form a small subset of breast cancers and it will be important to attempt to subdivide the larger group of tu-

Table 3. Prognosis and expression of basal and luminal markers

Antigen	Expressed in normal cells Basal	Luminal	Prognosis when expressed in cancers
PEM	-	++	Good *
ER	-	+/-	Good
VIMENTIN	+	-	Bad
KERATIN 14	+	-	Bad
EGF-R	++	+	Bad

* In a subset of tumours expressing extracellular mucin carrying an epitope expressed by the normally processed mucin

mours, which do not express basal markers and more closely resemble the luminal cell, into groups with good or bad prognosis. Expression of the oestrogen receptor defines one subgrouping. However, there are several other markers (not necessarily expressed by normal epithelial cells) which may be useful in this context.

Proliferative Potential of Luminal and Basal Cells from the Normal Breast *in Vitro*

Epithelial cells from the normal human mammary gland can be cultured either from tissue obtained at reduction mammoplasty (RM) surgery [53,54] or from milk [55,56]. The RM tissue contains both basal and luminal cells in the organoids, which can be separated from the fibroblasts, while the milk contains only luminal cells. Luminal cells can be cultured from milk using a complex serum containing medium (Milk Mix) but they have a limited *in vitro* life span [56]. Using the same medium, these cells can also be selectively cultured from RM tissue, again only for a few divisions [57]. Thus, the cell which *in vitro* shows the same antigenic profile as the luminal cells, has a poor proliferative potential. When RM organoids are cultured in a defined medium (MCDB170) containing pituitary extract instead of serum [58], the basal layer of cells grows out [57]. After a few passages, most of these cells senesce and a cell emerges which shows some of the properties of a stem cell, i.e., it has a high proliferative potential and expresses both basal and luminal keratins (not, however, keratin 19). This data suggests that there is a cell in the basal layer which has a high proliferative potential, which may give rise to cells showing features of the luminal epithelial cell phenotype. It is interesting that the cell which proliferates in long-term culture can express keratins 8 and 18 along with keratin 14, but keratin 19 is not expressed. (This keratin is, however, expressed in most of the luminal cells cultured from milk or from RM organoids in the alternative medium). Assuming that the keratin 19-negative luminal cell is precursor to the keratin 19-positive luminal cell, it appears that this last differentiation step is not induced in culture, but expression of keratin 19 is maintained in culture in those cells already expressing it *in vivo*. Figure 4 outlines a possible lineage suggested from this data, showing a cell in the basal layer giving rise to a keratin 19-negative luminal cell, which *in vivo* is precursor to the keratin 19-positive cell.

Phenotype of Cultured Breast Cancer Cell Lines

Breast Cancer Cell Lines

The immunohistochemical analysis of normal breast tissue and breast cancers suggested that the majority of cells in most of the carcinomas express antigens characteristic of the normal luminal epithelial cells, i.e., they express PEM, keratins 7, 8, 18 and 19 (sometimes ER) and do not express vimentin, keratin 14 or over-express EGF-R. The expression of the luminal markers appears to be extremely stable since several breast cancer cell lines which have been in culture for many years continue to express these antigens. Thus, most ER+ receptor-positive breast

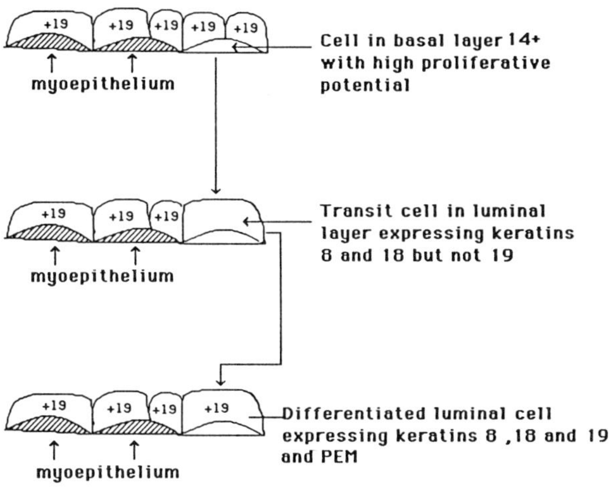

Fig. 4. Proposed scheme for development of luminal epithelial cell from a cell in the basal layer of the adult human mammary gland. Note: the phenotype of the **malignant** cell corresponds to that of the differentiated luminal epithelial cell

cancer cell lines (e.g., T47D, ZR75, MCF-7) and some oestrogen receptor-negative ones (eg. BT20) express keratins 8, 18 and 19 homogeneously and some also express keratin 7. These cells do not express keratin 14 and although the expression of vimentin remains controversial, most laboratories report that oestrogen receptor-positive cell lines do not express vimentin [57,59,60]. It is important to remember that most breast cancer cell lines in general use were developed from metastatic cells in serous effusions. In this case, when the cells are growing in suspension, Raemakers and colleagues [61] have shown that vimentin expression is readily induced. In fact, there are several cell lines, derived from breast cancers, which express vimentin [59]. All of these are oestrogen receptor-negative and could represent less differentiated cells which grew out from the carcinoma.

Cells Cultured from Primary Breast Cancers

It is notoriously difficult to culture demonstrably malignant cells from primary breast cancers. The most widely known cell line derived from this source is the oestrogen receptor-negative BT20. BT20 expresses keratins 8, 18 and 19 and has been found to be completely negative in its reaction with vimentin antibodies [J. Bartek, personal communication; 60]. Another cell line from a primary cancer, BT474, shows a similar profile of intermediate filament expression. Although there are several other lines reported in the literature to be derived from primary breast cancers, their intermediate filament expression has not been properly characterised.

The difficulty in obtaining cell lines from primary breast cancers indicates that the invasive cells in breast cancers are difficult to propagate. It is therefore crucial to use markers to examine the proliferating cells in short-term cultures. Antibodies to intermediate filament proteins along with other markers give some idea as to which cells are being propagated in different media. Using these criteria, the same cell type is found to proliferate in medium MCDB 170 as is seen in normal cell cultures, initially resembling the basal cell, then acquiring stem cell properties. This cell usually has a shorter life span than the cells cultured from normal tissue. Since the cells are diploid even when grown from aneuploid tumour [62], it seems likely that the cells cultured in this medium do not come from the invasive compartment. The shorter *in-vitro* life span could then be explained by the fact that only a fraction of the cells (non-malignant or pre-malignant) are proliferating.

The poor growth in culture of cells from the invasive component of primary breast cancers is in sharp contrast to the ability of these cells to metastasise and kill the patient. However, it has to be remembered that the *in vivo* progression of the disease can be very slow. Where the majority of tumour cells show the phenotype of the luminal cell, these may represent cells with a poor proliferative capacity which have arisen from a small compartment of less differentiated dividing cells. In this case we have to assume that the culture conditions do not favour the replacement type growth of this smaller compartment of cells: either they do not proliferate, or their progeny do not. Whatever happens *in vitro*, clearly cancer cells with the phenotype of the luminal cell can and do eventually proliferate and metastasise since many pleural effusion cell lines express this phenotype (see above).

There are several questions unanswered relating to the poor proliferative capacity of primary breast cancer cells. However, the observations do support the immunohistochemical data, and the observations on cultured normal cells, that the majority of breast cancer cells exhibit the luminal phenotype which has a low proliferative capacity *in vitro*. It will be of interest to see if it is easier to culture those tumours expressing the basal markers vimentin, keratin 14 or EGF-R, to see if they proliferate better. This would support the notion arising from the prognostic studies and the RM culture work that precursor cells with a high proliferative potential reside in the basal layer.

In attempting to assemble the facts regarding antigen expression, prognosis and proliferative capacity of breast cancer cells, the best fit is to assume that at least some of the changes leading to malignancy have occurred in a putative "stem" cell in the basal layer. Since, however, most of the cells in the carcinoma show the phenotype of the K19-positive luminal cell it is necessary to assume that the progeny of the "stem" cell retain differentiation potential, and eventually give rise to a large number of non-dividing cells, or cells with a very slow division rate. In fact, in those cases where cycle times have been measured in breast cancers, they are very high, particularly if compared to the impressive division potential of the mammary epithelial cells seen at pregnancy. This hypothesis would explain why it is so difficult to culture primary breast cancer cells. It also allows for the possibility that in those tumours which express basal markers, there is a larger component of proliferating precursor cells, which would be responsible for the poor prognosis associated with these tumours.

A problem arises in resolving how a cell type which apparently has poor proliferative potential in the primary tumour invades, metastasises and proliferates. This must be the case since the phenotype of many cell lines derived from metastases corresponds to that of the keratin 19-positive luminal cell. As indicated earlier, the time factor involved in the step from primary tumour to metastasis has to be considered in trying to explain this change. Where the luminal phenotype is maintained, we have to assume that the cell slowly acquires division potential, or possibly is stimulated to grow by other factors in the metastatic site. Where the basal markers (e.g., vimentin) appear, it is likely that a shift occurs so that the more primitive precursor compartment with a higher growth rate is enlarged. I have attempted to outline these highly speculative ideas (see Fig. 4) mainly to provide a framework for thinking about the problem and for planning other experiments. There are some obvious studies which should be done. For example, the relation between keratin 19 expression and prognosis should be examined. Also, a more complete analysis of the expression of all the basal markers in a series of tumours needs to be done. Finally, detailed definition of the phenotype of a wide range of breast cancer cell lines is required, and attempts made to relate the phenotype and *in-vitro* growth potential of primary and metastatic lesions from the same patient.

Conclusion and Discussion

The definition of the malignant phenotype in terms of the normal cell lineage is important for a variety of reasons (see Table 4). Here I have emphasised the use of differentiation antigens and antibodies to them as prognostic indicators. However, there are wider impli-

Table 4. Importance of defining malignant phenotype in terms of the normal cell lineage

1	May identify highly or less highly differentiated tumours and predict prognosis
2	Identify tumour-associated antigens (targets for McAbs and possible immunogens)
3	For comparisons of normal and malignant cells it is necessary to identify differences associated with malignancy and therefore there is a need to compare appropriate cells
4	To know which normal cells to culture in order to examine the effects of oncogenes and growth factors thought to be related to breast cancer

cations for knowing exactly which cell in the normal cell lineage the malignant cell is to be compared to. Without this definition comparisons relating to malignancy cannot be made. With this definition it is possible to take a more meaningful approach to developing culture systems for the appropriate normal cells to investigate the effects of factors thought to be involved in breast cancer. Moreover, although the culture of malignant cells from primary breast cancers remains a problem, this approach at least allows the careful definition of the phenotype of the cells which proliferate in short-term culture. While studies on patients are clearly crucial, they are slow. It is therefore highly desirable to back them up with studies in experimental systems which can be manipulated *in vitro*. In these systems it is essential to know the cells we are or should be dealing with, and it is therefore crucial that the definition of cell phenotypes needs be pursued.

REFERENCES

1 Taylor-Papadimitrou J and Gendler SJ: Molecular aspects of mucins. In: Hilgers J and Zotter S (eds) Cancer Reviews Vol. 11-12, Munksgaard, Copenhagen, Denmark 1988 pp 11-24

2 Gendler S, Taylor-Papadimitriou J, Burchell J and Duhig T: A polymorphic epithelial mucin expressed by breast and other carcinomas: Immunological and molecular studies. In: Human Tumor Antigens and Specific Tumor Therapy, UCLA Symposia on Molecular and Cellular Biology, New Series, Vol 99, Alan R Liss, Inc, New York 1989 pp 11-23

3 Gendler SJ, Lancaster CA, Taylor-Papadimitriou J, Duhig T, Peat N, Burchell J, Pemberton L, Lalani E-N and Wilson D: Molecular cloning and expression of the human tumour-associated polymorphic epithelial mucin. J Biol Chem 1990 (265):15286-15293

4 Lancaster CA, Peat N, Duhig T, Wilson D, Taylor-Papadimitiou J and Gendler SJ: Structure and expression of PEM: a gene conserving methylated CpGs in an expressed VNTR unit. Biochem Biophys Res Commun 1990 (173):1019-1029

5 Wreschner DH, Hareuveni M, Tsarfaty I et al: Human epithelial tumor antigen cDNA sequences. Eur J Biochem 1990 (189):463-473

6 Siddiqui J, Abe M, Hayes D, Shani E, Yunis E and Kufe D: Isolation and sequencing of a cDNA coding for the human DF3 breast carcinoma-associated antigen. Proc Natl Acad Sci USA 1990 (85):2320-2323

7 Ligtenberg M, Vos H, Gennissen A and Hilkens J: Episialin, a carcinoma-associated mucin, is generated by a polymorphic gene encoding splice variants with alternative amino termini. J Biol Chem 1990 (265):5573-5578

8 Swallow DM, Gendler S, Griffiths B, Corney G, Taylor-Papadimitriou J and Bramwell ME: The human tumour-associated epithelial mucins are coded by an expressed hypervariable gene locus PUM. Nature 1987 (328):82-84

9 Girling A, Bartkova J, Burchell J, Gendler S, Gillett C and Taylor-Papadimitriou J: A core protein epitope of the polymorphic epithelial mucin detected by the monoclonal antibody SM-3 is selectively exposed in a range of primary carcinomas. Int J Cancer 1989 (43):1072-1076

10 Hull SR, Bright A, Carraway KL, Abe M and Kufe D: Oligosaccharides of the DF3 antigen of the BT20 human breast carcinoma cell line. J Cell Biochem 1988 (Suppl 12E):130, Abstract

11 Hanisch F-G, Uhlenbruck G, Peter-Katalinic J, Egge H, Dabrowski J and Dabrowski U: Structures of neutral O-linked polylactosaminoglycans on human skim milk mucins. A novel type of linearly extended poly-N-acetyl-lactosamine backbones with Gal 3b(1-4) GlcNAc 3b(1-6) repeating units. J Biol Chem 1989 (264):872-883

12 Burchell J, Gendler S, Taylor-Papadimitriou J, Girling A, Lewis A, Millis R and Lamport D: Development and characterisation of breast cancer reactive monoclonal antibodies directed to the core protein of the human milk mucin. Cancer Res 1987 (47):5476-5482

13 Jerome KR, Barnd DL, Bendt KM, Boyer CM, Taylor-Papadimitriou J, McKenzie IFC, Bast RC, Jr and Finn OJ: Cytotoxic T-lymphocytes derived from patients with breast adenocarcinoma recognize an epitope present on the protein core of a mucin molecule preferentially expressed by malignant cells. Cancer Res 1991 (51):2908-2916

14 Granowska M, Mather SJ, Jobling T, Naeem M, Burchell J, Taylor-Papadimitriou J, Shepherd J and Britton KE: Radiolabelled stripped mucin, SM3, monoclonal antibody for immunoscintigraphy of ovarian tumours. Int J Biol Mark 1990 (5):89-96

15 Wilkinson MJS, Howell A, Harris M, Taylor-Papadimitriou J, Swindell R and Sellwood RA: The prognostic significance of two epithelial membrane antigens expressed by human mammary carcinomas. Int J Cancer 1984 (33):299-304

16 Nagle RB: Intermediate filaments: A review of the basic biology. Am J Surg Pathol 1988 (12):4-16

17 Moll R, Franke WW, Schiller DL, Geiger B and Krepler R: The catalog of human cytokeratins: patterns of expression of specific cytokeratins in normal epithelia, tumors and cultured cells. Cell 1982 (31):11-24

18 Moll R, Schiller DLK and Franke WW: Identification of protein IT of the intestinal cytoskeleton as a novel Type I cytokeratin with unusual properties and expression patterns. J Cell Biol 1990 (111): 567-579

19 Guelstein VI, Tchpysheva TA, Ermilova VD, Litvinova LV, Troyanovsky SM and Bannikov GA: Monoclonal antibody mapping of keratins 8 and 17 and of vimentin in normal human mammary gland, benign tumors, dysplasias and breast cancer. Int J Cancer 1988 (42): 147-153

20 Taylor-Papadimitriou J, Wetzels R and Ramaekers F: Intermediate filament protein expression in normal and malignant human mammary epithelial cells. In: Dickson RB and Lippman ME (eds) Breast Cancer: Cellular and Molecular Biology III. Kluwer 1991 (in press)

21 Gould VE, Koukoulis GK, Jansson DS, Nagle RB, Franke WW and Moll R: Coexpression patterns of vimentin and glial filament protein with cytokeratins

in the normal, hyperplastic, and neoplastic breast. Am J Pathol 1990 (137):1143-1155

22 Nagle RB, Boecker W, Davis JR, Heid HW, Kaufmann M, Lucas DO and Jarasch E-D: Characterisation of breast carcinomas by two monoclonal antibodies distinguishing myoepithelial from luminal epithelial cells. J Histochem Cytochem 1986 (34):869-881

23 Bartek J, Durban EM, Hallowes RC and Taylor-Papadimitriou J: A subclass of luminal epithelial cells in the human mammary gland, defined by antibodies to cytokeratins. J Cell Sci 1985 (75):17-33

24 Bartek J, Bartkova J and Taylor-Papadimitriou J: Keratin 19 expression in the adult and developing human mammary gland. Histochem J 1990 (22):537-544

25 Bartek J, Taylor-Papadimitriou J, Miller N and Millis R: Patterns of expression of keratin 19 as detected with monoclonal antibodies in human breast tissues and tumours. Int J Cancer 1985 (36):299-306

26 Bartek J, Bartkova J, Schneider J, Taylor-Papadimitriou J, Kovarik J and Rejthar A: Expression of monoclonal antibody-defined epitopes of keratin 19 in human tumours and cultured cells. Eur J Cancer Clin Oncol 1986 (32):1441-1452

27 Azumi N and Battifora H: The distribution of vimentin and keratin in epithelial and nonepithelial neoplasms. Am J Clin Pathol 1987 (88):286

28 Raymond WA and Leong A S-Y: Co-expression of cytokeratin and vimentin intermediate filament proteins in benign and neoplastic breast epithelium. J Pathol 1989 (157):299-306

29 Cattoretti G, Andreola S, Clemente, C, D'Amato L and Rilke F: Vimentin and p53 expression in epidermal growth factor receptor-positive, oestrogen receptor-negative breast carcinomas. Br J Cancer 1988 (57):353-357

30 Domagala W, Wozniak L, Lasota J, Weber K and Osborn M: Vimentin is preferentially expressed in high-grade ductal and medullary, but not in lobular breast carcinomas. Am J Pathol 1990 (137):1059-1064

31 Raymond WA and Leong ASY: Vimentin - A new prognostic parameter in breast carcinoma. J Pathol 1989 (158):107-114

32 Domagala W, Lasota J, Bartkowiak J, Weber K and Osborn M: Vimentin is preferentially expressed in human breast carcinomas with low estrogen receptor and high Ki-67 growth fraction. Am J Pathol 1990 (136):219-227

33 Domagala W, Lasota J, Dukowicz A, Markiewski M, Striker G, Weber K and Osborn M: Vimentin expression appears to be associated with poor prognosis in node-negative ductal NOS breast carcinomas. Am J Pathol 1990 (137):1299-1304

34 Dairkee HS, Puett L and Hackett, AJ: Expression of basal and luminal epithelium-specific keratins in normal, benign and malignant breast tissue. JNCI 1988 (80):691-695

35 Wetzels RHW, Holland R, van Haelst UJGM, Lane EB, Leigh IM and Ramaekers FCS: Detection of basement membrane components and basal cell keratin 14 in noninvasive and invasive carinomas of the breast. Am J Pathol 1990 (134):571-579

36 Dairkee SH, Mayall BH, Smith HS: Monoclonal marker that predicts early recurrence of breast cancer. Lancet 1987 (1):514-516

37 Slamon DJ, Clark GM, Wong SG, Levin WJ, Ullrich A, McGuire WL: Amplification of the her-2/neu oncogene correlates with relapse and survival in human cancer. Science 1987 (235):177-182

38 van de Vijver, Peterse JL, Mooi WJ, Wisman P, Lomans J, Dalesio O, and Nusse R: Neu-protein overexpression in breast cancer. Association with the comedo type ductal carcinoma in situ and limited prognostic value in stage II breast cancer. N Engl J Med 1988 (319):1239-1245

39 Meissner K, Riviere A, Haupt G and Loning T: Study of Neu-protein expression in mammary Paget's disease with and without underlying breast carcinoma and in extramammary Paget's disease. Am J Pathol 1990 (137):1305-1309

40 Jacquemier JD, Hassoun J, Torrente M and Martin P-M: Districution of estrogen and progesterone receptors in healthy tissue adjacent to breast lesions in various stages - Immunohistochemical study of 107 cases. Breast Cancer Res and Treat 1990 (15): 109-117

41 Petersen OW, Hoyer PE and van Deurs B: Frequency and distribution of estrogen receptor-positive cells in normal, nonlactating human breast tissue. Cancer Res 1987 (47): 5748-5751

42 Battersby S, Robertson BJ Anderson TJ, King RJB and McPherson K: Influence of menstrual cycle, parity and oral contraceptive use on steroid hormone receptos in normal breast. 1991 (in press)

43 Perez R, Pascual M, Macias A and Lage A: Epidermal growth factor receptos in human breast cancer. Breast Cancer Res Treat 1984 (4): 189-193

44 Fitzpatrick SL, Brightwell J, Wittliff JL, Barrows GH and Schultz GS: Epidermal growth factor binding by breast-tumour biopsies and relationship to estrogen receptor and progestin receptor levels. Cancer Res 1984 (44): 3448-3453

45 Sainsbury JRC, Farndon JJ, Sherbet GV and Harris AL: Epidermal-growth-factor receptors and

oestrogen receptors in human breast cancer. Lancet 1985 (i): 364-366

46 Nicholson S, Sainsbury JRC, Halcrow P, Chambers P, Farndon JR and Harris AL: Expression of epidermal-growth-factor receptors associated with lack of response to endocrine therapy in recurrent breast cancer. Lancet 1989 (i): 182-185

47 Sainsbury JRC, Farndon JR, Needham GK, Malcolm AJ, Harris AL: Epidermal growth factor receptor status as predictor of early recurrence and death from breast cancer. Lancet 1987 (i): 1982-1987

48 Tsutsumi Y, Naber SP, deLellis RA, Wolfe HJ, Marks PJ, McKenzie SJ and Yin S: Neu oncogene protein and epidermal growth factor receptor are independently expressed in benign and malignant breast tissues. Hum Pathol 1990 (21): 750-758

49 Stoker MGP, Pigott D and Taylor-Papadimitriou J: Response to epidermal growth factors of cultured human mammary epithelial cells from benign tumours. Nature 1976 (39): 279-282

50 Taylor-Papadimitriou J, Shearer M and Stoker MGP: Growth requirements of human mammary cells in culture. Int J Cancer 1977 (20):903-908

51 Snedeker SM, Brown CF, DiAugstine RP: Expression and functional properties of transforming growth factor 3a and epidermal growth factor during mouse mammary gland ductal morphogenesis. Proc Natl Acad Sci USA 1991 (88): 276-280

52 Valverius EM, Velu T, Shakar V, Ciardiello F, Kim N and Salomon DS: Over-expression of the epidermal growth factor receptor in human breast cancer cells fails to induce an estrogen-independent phenotype. Int J Cancer 1990 (46): 712-718

53 Stampfer M. Hallowes RC and Hackett AJ: Growth of normal human mammary cells in culture. In Vitro 1980 (16): 415-425

54 Stampfer MR: Cholera toxin stimulation of human mammary epithelial cells in culture. In Vitro 1982 (18):531-537

55 Buehring GC: Culture of human mammary epithelial cells: Keeping abreast of a new method. J Natl Cancer Inst 1972 (49): 1433-1434

56 Taylor-Papadimitrou J, Purkis P and Fentiman IS: Cholera toxia and analogues of cyclic AMP stimulate the growth of cultured mammary epithelial cells. J Cell Physiol 1980 (102): 317-321

57 Taylor-Papadimitrou J, Stampfer M, Bartek J, Lewis A, Boshell M, Lane EB and Leigh IM: Keratin expression in human mammary epithelial cells cultured from normal and malignant tissue: relation to in vivo phenotypes and influence of medium. J Cell Science 1989 (94): 403-413

58 Hammond SL, Ham RG and Stmpfer MR: Serum-free growth of human mammary epithelial cells: Rapid clonal growth in defined medium and extended serial passage with pituitary extract. Proc Natl Acad Sci USA 1984 (81): 5435-5439

59 Sommers CL, Walker-Jones D, Heckford SE, Worland P, Valverius E, Clark R, McCormick F, Stampfer M, Abularach S and Gelmann EP: Vimentin rather than keratin expression in some hormone-independent breast cancer cell lines and in oncogene-transformed mammary epithelial cells. Cancer Res 1989 (49):4258-4263

60 Curschellas E, Matter A and Regenass U: Immunolocalization of cytoskeletal elements in human mammary epithelial cells. Eur J Cancer Clin Oncol 1987 (23):1517-1527

61 Ramaekers FCS, Haag D, Kant A, Moesker O, Jap PHK and Vooijs GP: Coexpression of keratin and vimentin-type intermediate filaments in human metastatic carcinoma cells. Proc Natl Acad Sci USA 1983 (80):2618-2622

62 Wolman SR, Smith HS, Stampfer M and Hackett AJ: Growth of diploid cells from breast cancers. Cancer Genet Cytogenet 1985 (16):49-64

The Oestrogen-Regulated pS_2-BCEI Protein in Breast Cancer

Edwin Milgrom

Unité INSERM U. 135, Hôpital de Bicêtre, Le Kremlin Bicêtre, France

About one-third of patients with advanced breast cancer respond to hormone therapy [1]. Adequate prescription of this treatment is, therefore, required to devise means of predicting their response. Oestrogen receptor determinations have proved to be effective in this respect: receptor-negative patients displayed remission in less than 5-10% of cases, whereas remission was observed in ~50% of ER-positive patients. In order to improve this prediction, a search was made for efficient markers of oestrogen action. One of these is the oestrogen-inducible progesterone receptor: ER+ PR+ patients have ~75% probability to respond to hormone therapy. Also other oestrogen-responsive markers have been defined, for example, Cathepsin D [2]. Random cloning of oestrogen-responsive messenger RNAs was performed independently by 2 groups [3-5]. It allowed to define a messenger RNA called pS_2 or BCEI (Breast Cancer Oestrogen Induced), which has been extensively characterised. It was studied not only as a means of predicting response to hormone therapy in advanced breast cancer, but also as a predictor of outcome in early cancer and as a model of oestrogen regulation of a human target gene.

Cloning of a DNA Complementary to pS_2-BCEI Messenger RNA [3]

A cDNA library was set up with messenger RNAs prepared from oestrogen-treated MCF-7 breast cancer cells. The clones were screened with 2 probe preparations: one consisted of DNAs complementary to messenger RNAs from oestrogen-treated cells, the other of DNAs complementary to messenger RNAs from non-treated cells. Such a differential hybridisation method yielded clones corresponding to messenger RNAs either induced or repressed by oestrogen. Among the former, one clone corresponded to a small (~600 nucleotides), relatively abundant (0.8% of the transcripts in oestrogen-treated MCF-7 cells) and strongly oestrogen-stimulated messenger RNA.
The same messenger RNA was subsequently cloned by Westley and collaborators who analysed oestrogen-induced messenger RNAs in different breast cancer cell types [6].

Structure and Putative Function of the pS_2/BCEI Protein

The sequencing of the cloned cDNA revealed an 84 amino-acid long open reading frame. A signal peptide suggested that the protein was secreted from the cell [3,4]. Subsequently, the protein was isolated from MCF-7 culture media and partially sequenced [7,8]. It was observed that the N-terminal amino acid was a glutamic acid and that the mature protein after excision of the signal peptide thus consisted of 60 amino acids. The small size and a very peculiar arrangement of disulphide bonds were similar to those of some growth factors [3]. However, initial searches in the data banks did not show any homology with known proteins.
It was only in 1988 that Baker [9] observed the homology between pS_2 and pancreatic spasmophilic polypeptide (PSP). The latter is

a protein of 106 amino acids (molecular weight 11,700 Da), which modulates the mobility of the gastro-intestinal tract and regulates gastric acid secretion [10,11]. When the mechanism of action of PSP was studied [12], specific receptors were detected in the gastro-intestinal tract and an inhibition of the synthesis of cAMP was observed in membranes of mucosal intestinal cells [13]. The human and murine equivalents of porcine PSP have been cloned [14]. This analogy of pS_2 with PSP suggests that they may have similar mechanisms of action but at present no data are available on the biological activity of pS_2.

Hormonal Regulation of pS_2

Initial studies [3] showed the specificity of regulation of pS_2 messenger RNA by oestrogens: no effect was observed with glucocorticoids, progestin and androgen. This was further confirmed by the very low concentration of oestradiol (0.05 nM) sufficient to elicit half the maximal induction of pS_2 messenger RNA.

Many studies have been dedicated to antioestrogen effects on pS_2 messenger RNA concentration. It was confirmed that tamoxifen and hydroxytamoxifen are complete antagonists (as they are for Cathepsin D induction), whereas in the same MCF7 cells they are partial agonists when considering progesterone receptor concentration or its messenger RNA [15-20]. In order to analyse the possible involvement of pS_2 in oestrogen growth promoting effects, various antioestrogen-resistant cell line variants were studied. Davidson et al. [21] showed in 2 variants of MCF-7 (I13 and LY12) that antioestrogen and oestrogen effects on growth were not correlated with pS_2 messenger RNA (and Cathepsin D) variations. They concluded that these proteins were not major autocrine factors controlling the growth of breast cancer cells. Similar conclusions were reached by other groups [22,23].

Modulation of pS_2 messenger RNA was also observed under the effect of various growth factors (EGF, insulin, IGF, basic FGF). However, these effects appeared to be secondary and indirect, as opposed to pS_2 messenger RNA induction by oestrogen [24].

Further studies were undertaken by Chambon and collaborators at the level of the gene [25].

The oestrogen-responsive element (ERE) was localised upstream of the transcription starting site [26] and further identified [27] as an imperfect 13 bp palindrome localised at position -405 -393 of the gene. This ERE diverges by 1 base from the canonical perfect palindromic ERE.

Responsive elements to phorbol esters (activators of Protein kinase C), EGF, c-Haras and c-jun proteins were also present in the region -428 to -332 [28]. Thus, the effect of oestrogen on pS_2 gene transcription was probably double: direct on the ERE through the oestrogen receptor, indirect through oestrogen-induced activation of various growth-responsive genes which in turn activate the pS_2 promoter [28]. Transgenic mice expressing pS_2 in breast and secreting it into milk were also produced [29].

The gene encoding pS_2 protein was localised to human chromosome 21 [30]. It was shown that the gene was neither amplified nor grossly modified in MCF-cells [3].

Cellular Distribution of pS_2 Messenger RNA and Protein

It was initially suggested that pS_2 expression was restricted to malignant breast cancer cells and was absent in normal breast tissue and in benign tumours [31,32]. However, further studies argued against this hypothesis: pS_2 mRNA was detected in some fibroadenomas [3]. This was recently confirmed by using a sensitive ELISA assay [33]. The mean concentration of pS_2 in normal breast tissue was 0.48 ng/mg of protein, in benign breast tumours it was 1.71 ng/mg protein and in breast cancers 10.4 ng/mg protein. pS_2 was also detected in normal breast tissue and benign tumours by immunohistochemistry [34].

Westley and collaborators analysed the presence of pS_2 messenger RNA in different breast cancer cells lines: besides in MCF-7 it was also found in a relatively high concentra-

tion in ZR-75 but its concentration was very low in T47-D cells [6,35].
Chambon and collaborators [36] identified the protein and its mRNA in normal gastric tissue and found similar concentrations in men and women. The protein was also present in gastric secretion. In a more extensive study [37], pS_2 messenger RNA was found in all the 75 biopsies of normal stomach while it was only present in a fraction (67%) of gastric cancers. pS_2 messenger RNA was absent in well differentiated gastric cancer cell lines, contrarily to the poorly differentiated cell lines. pS_2 messenger RNA was also detected in other cancer types: 6/29 ovarian cancers, 2/55 endometrial carcinomas and 2/33 cervical cancers [38-40].

Antibodies to pS_2 and Assay Methods

Both polyclonal and monoclonal antibodies have been developed [41-43]. Prud'homme et al. [44] expressed the protein in E. coli in fusion with ß galactosidase. After immunisation of mice, a panel of hybridoma cell lines secreting anti-pS_2 antibodies was characterised. It was observed that the monoclonals belonged to 2 categories: preferentially recognising either the denatured form of the protein or its native form. Among the latter a very high affinity monoclonal antibody was obtained which could be used at low concentration (2 µg/ml) for immunohistochemistry on both frozen and paraffin embedded sections (Fig. 1). The same antibody could be used for one-step immunoaffinity purification of the protein (Fig. 2).
An immunoradiometric method [42] and an immunoenzymatic ELISA method [33] were developed for the assay of pS_2 in breast tumour extracts. The ELISA method was of sufficient sensitivity (1.8 pg/ml) to allow to measure the amount of the protein in blood (M.F. Pichon et al., manuscript in preparation).

Assay of pS_2 as a Means of Outcome Prediction in Breast Cancer

Foekens et al. [42] used the IRMA method to assay the cytosolic levels of pS_2 in a bank of 205 breast cancer fragments, while Predine et al. [33] used the ELISA assay to perform similar measurements on 339 breast cancers. Both groups observed that pS_2 concentration was not correlated with tumour size and lymph-node status.
Only Predine et al. [33] reported a correlation with menopausal status (higher concentration in premenopausal women) and differentiation (lower concentration in grade III tumours). In both studies a strong correlation was found with the presence of oestrogen and progesterone receptors.
Foekens et al. [42], using a cutoff of 11 ng of pS_2/mg of cytosolic protein, observed a strong correlation with relapse-free survival and overall survival. For instance, the death rate for patients with pS_2^+ tumours (27 % of the patients) was one-tenth of the death rate

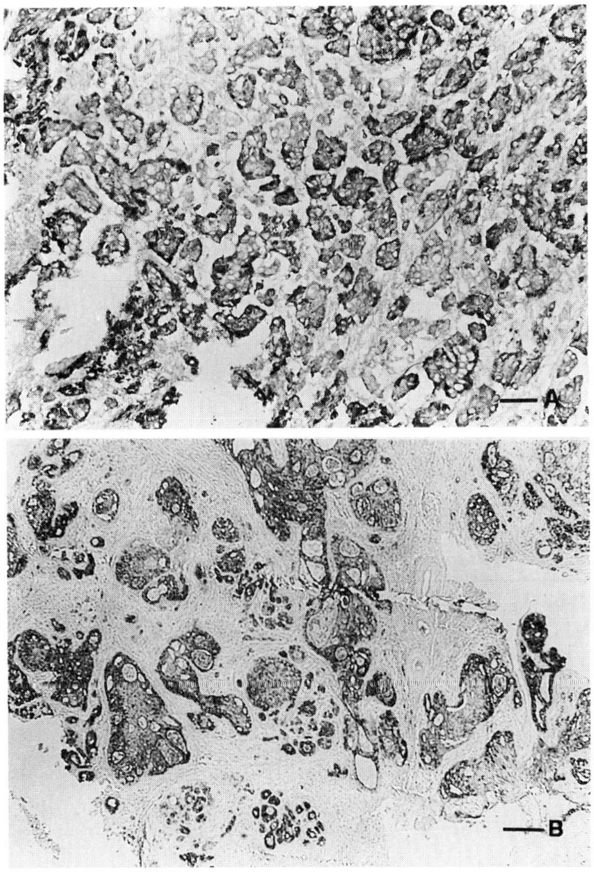

Fig. 1. Immunocytochemical detection of pS_2 in human breast cancer
A - Frozen section
B - Paraffin embedded section

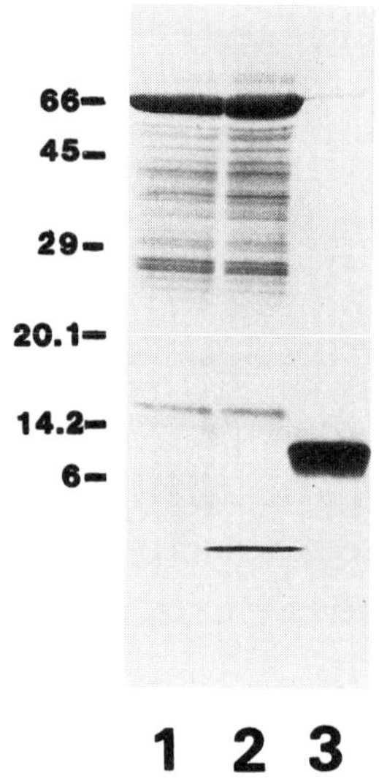

Fig. 2. One step immunoaffinity purification of pS_2
Cell culture medium was obtained from oestrogen-treated MCF-7 cells. It was chromatographed on a $mBCEI_{11}$-$Affigel_{10}$ column.
Polyacrylamide (15%) gel electrophoresis in the presence of sodium dodecyl sulphate:
lane 1: culture medium from the MCF-7 cells
lane 2: flow-through of immunoaffinity chromatography column
lane 3: protein eluted from the immunomatrix

for patients with pS_2^- ER^- tumours. These authors also concluded that knowledge of the cytosolic pS_2 status was of particular importance to identify patients at high risk in the ER^+/PgR^+ subclass of tumours and in both the N0 and N+ subclasses of patients.
Largely different results were obtained by Predine et al. [33] who concluded that the prognostic value of pS_2 determinations was rather limited.
Using the same cutoff point as Foekens et al. [42] or isolating the 1/4 or 1/3 of patients having the highest concentration of pS_2 did not allow to observe a statistically significant correlation with disease-free interval or overall survival. In this study the prognostic value of pS_2 was only apparent for a relatively small group of patients (15%) who had low values of pS_2 ($\leq$ 0.32 ng/mg of protein). These patients had a shorter disease-free interval and overall survival.
The reasons for these discrepancies are not clearly understood. They may be due to differences in methodology (for instance the sensitivity of the ELISA method allowing measurements of low levels of pS_2), or to differences in patient characteristics. The group studied by Foekens et al. [42] showed an unusual proportion of bad prognosis patients (see discussion in [33]).
Predine et al. [33] observed that pS_2 concentration was very strongly correlated with the outcome of adjuvant hormone therapy. They observed that in multivariate analysis pS_2 appeared the most powerful factor for predicting disease-free as well as overall survival in patients receiving tamoxifen, even preceding the well established oestrogen receptor determination. Schwartz et al. [45] recently observed that pS_2 expression may define a subset of ER-positive tumours that are more likely to respond to hormonal treatment.
Further studies including large numbers of patients will be necessary to accurately determine the value of pS_2 determinations in defining the prognosis of primary breast cancer and in predicting the outcome of endocrine therapies.

Acknowledgments

J. F. Prud'homme has done most of the experiments on pS_2-BCEI performed in our laboratory.
This work was supported by the INSERM, the UFR Kremlin-Bicêtre, the Fondation pour la Recherche Médicale Française, the Association pour la Recherche sur le Cancer and Transbio Company.
M. Guerrois and V. Marie typed the manuscript.

REFERENCES

1 Santen RJ, Manni A, Harvey H and Redmond C: Endocrine treatment of breast cancer in women. Endocr Rev 1990 (11):221-265

2 Rochefort H: Cathepsin D in breast cancer. Breast Cancer Res Treat 1990 (16):1-13

3 Prud'homme JF, Fridlansky F, Le Cunff M, Atger M, Mercier Bodart C, Pichon MF and Milgrom E: Cloning of a gene expressed in human breast cancer and regulated by estrogen in MCF-7 cells. DNA 1985 (4):11-21

4 Jakowlew SB, Breathnach R, Jeltsch JM, Masiakowski P and Chambon P: Sequence of the pS2 mRNA induced by estrogen in the human breast cancer cell line MCF7. Nucl Acid Res 1984 (12):2861-2878

5 Masiakowski P, Breathnach R, Bloch J, Gannon F, Krust A and Chambon P: Cloning of cDNA sequences of hormone regulated genes from the MCF7 human breast cancer cell line. Nucl Acid Res 1982 (10):7895-7901

6 May FEB and Westley BR: Identification and characterization of estrogen regulated RNAs in human breast cancer cells. J Biol Chem 1988 (263):12901-12908

7 Rio MC, Lepage P, Diemunsch P, Roitsch C and Chambon P: Structure primaire de la proteine humaine pS2. CR Acad Sci III Paris 1988 (307):825-831

8 Mori K, Fujii R, Kida N, Ohta M and Hayashi K: Identification of a polypeptide secreted by human breast cancer cells (MCF7) as the human estrogen responsive gene (pS2) product. Biochem Biophys Res Commun 1988 (155):366-372

9 Baker EM: Oestrogen induced pS2 protein is similar to pancreatic spasmolytic polypeptide and the kringle domain. Biochem J 1988 (253):307-311

10 Jorgensen KH, Thim L and Jacobsen HE: Pancreatic spasmolytic polypeptide (PSP): Preparation and initial chemical characterization of a new polypeptide from porcine pancreas. Regul Pept 1982 (3):207-219

11 Jorgensen KD, Diamant B, Jorgensen KH and Thim L: Pancreatic spasmolytic polypeptide (PSP): Pharmacology of a new porcine pancreatic polypeptide with spasmolytic and gastric acid secretion inhibitory effects. Regul Pept 1982 (3):231-243

12 Hoosein NM, Thim L, Jorgensen KH and Brattain MG: Growth stimulatory effect of pancreatic spasmolytic polypeptide on cultured colon and breast tumor cells. FEBS Lett 1989 (247):303-306

13 Frandsen EK, Jorgensen KH and Thim L: Receptor binding of pancreatic spasmolytic polypeptide (PSP) in rat intestinal mucosal cell membranes inhibits the adenylate cyclase activity. Regul Pept 1986 (16):291-297

14 Tomasetto C, Rio MC, Gautier C, Wolf C, Hareuveni M, Chambon P and Lathe R: hSP, the domain duplicated homolog pf pS2 protein, is co expressed with pS2 in stomach but not in breast carcinoma. Embo J 1990 (9):407-414

15 Weaver CA, Springer PA and Katzenellenbogen BS: Regulation of pS2 gene expression by affinity labeling and reversibly binding estrogens and antiestrogens: comparison of effects on the native gene and on pS2 chloramphenicol acetyltransferase fusion genes transfected into MCF7 human breast cancer cells. Mol Endocrinol 1988 (2):936-945

16 May FEB and Westley BR: Effects of tamoxifen and 4 hydroxytamoxifen on the pNR 1 and pNR 2 estrogen regulated RNAs in human breast cancer cells. J Biol Chem 1987 (262):15894-15899

17 Westley BR, Hölzel F and May FEB: Effects of oestrogen and the antioestrogens, tamoxifen and LY117018, on four oestrogen regulated RNAs in the EFM-19 breast cancer cell line. J Steroid Biochem 1989 (32):365-372

18 Kida N, Yoshimura T, Mori K and Hayashi K: Hormonal regulation of synthesis and secretion of pS2 protein relevant to growth of human breast cancer cells MCF7. Cancer Res 1989 (49):3494-3498

19 Henry JA, Nicholson S, Hennessy, Lennard TWJ, May FEB and Westley BR: Expression of the oestrogen regulated pNR2 mRNA in human breast cancer: relation to oestrogen receptor mRNA levels and response to tamoxifen therapy. Br J Cancer 1989 (61):32-38

20 Pilat MJ, Hafner M and Brooks SC: Differential induction of pS2 and Cathepsin D mRNAs by structurally altered estrogens. The Endocrine Society 1991 p 270

21 Davidson NE, Bronzert DA, Chambon P Gelmann EP and Lippman ME: Use of two MCF7 cell variants to evaluate the growth regulatory potential of estrogen induced products. Cancer Res 1986 (46):1904-1908

22 Westley B, May FEB, Brown AMC, Krust A, Chambon P, Lippman ME and Rochefort H: Effects of antiestrogens on the estrogen-regulated pS2 RNA and the 52- and 160-kilodalton proteins in MCF-7 cells and two tamoxifen-resistant sublines. J Biol Chem 1984 (259):10030-10035

23 Aitken SC, Lippman ME, Kasid A and Schoenberg DR: Relationship between the expression of estrogen regulated genes and estrogen stimulated proliferation of MCF7 mammary tumor cells. Cancer Res 1985 (45):2608-2615

24 Cavailles V, Garcia M and Rochefort H: Regulation of cathepsin D and pS2 gene expression by growth factors in MCF7 human breast cancer cells. Mol Endocrinol 1989 (3):552-558

25 Brown AMC, Jeltsch JM, Roberts M and Chambon P: Activation of pS2 gene transcription is a primary response to estrogen in the human breast cancer cell line MCF-7. Proc Natl Acad Sci USA 1984 pp 6344-6348

26 Roberts M, Wallace J, Jeltsch JM and Berry M: The 5' flanking region of the human pS2 gene mediates its transcriptional activation by estrogen in MCF7 cells. Biochem Biophys Res Commun 1988 (151):306-313

27 Berry M, Nunez AM and Chambon P: Estrogen responsive element of the human pS2 gene is an imperfectly palindromic sequence. Proc Natl Acad Sci USA 1986 pp 1218-1222

28 Nunez AM, Berry M, Imler JL and Chambon P: The 5' flanking region of the pS2 gene contains a complex enhancer region responsive to oestrogens, epidermal growth factor, a tumor promoter (TPA), the c-Ha-ras oncoprotein and the c-jun protein. Embo J 1989 (8):823-829
29 Tomasetto C, Wolf C, Rio MC, Mehtali M, LeMeur M, Gerlinger P, Chambon P and Lathe R: Breast cancer protein pS2 synthesis in mammary gland of transgenic mice and secretion into milk. Mol Endocrinol 1989 (3):1579-1584
30 Cohen Haguenauer O, Nguyen Van Cong, Prud'homme JF, Jegou-Joubert C, Gross MS, De Tand MF, Milgrom E and Frézal J: A gene expressed in human breast cancer and regulated by estrogen in MCF7 cells is located on chromosome 21. Eighth International Workshop on Human Gene Mapping 1985
(40) p 606
31 Rio MC, Bellocq JP, Gairard B, Koehl C, Renaud R and Chambon P: Expression spécifique du gène humain pS2 dans les cancers du sein. Biochimie 1988 (70):961-968
32 Rio MC and Chambon P: The pS2 gene, mRNA, and protein : a potential marker for the human breast cancer. Cancer Cells 1990 (2):269-274
33 Prédine J, Spyratos F, Prud'homme JF, Andrieu C, Hacene K, Brunet M, Pallud C and Milgrom E: Enzyme linked immunosorbent assay (ELISA) of pS2 in breast cancers, benign tumors and normal breast tissues. Correlation with prognosis and adjuvant hormonotherapy. Cancer (in press)
34 Pallud C, Le Doussal V, Pichon MF, Prud'homme JF, Hacene K and Milgrom E: Immunohistochemistry of pS2 in normal human breast cancer and in various histological forms of breast tumors. Submitted for publication
35 May FEB and Westley BR: Cloning of estrogen regulated messenger RNA sequences from human breast cancer cells. Cancer Res 1986 (46):6034-6040
36 Rio MC, Bellocq JP, Daniel JY, Tomasetto C, Lathe R, Chenard MP, Batzenschaler A and Chambon P: Breast cancer associated pS2 protein: synthesis and secretion by normal stomach mucosa. Science 1988 (241):705-708
37 Luqmani Y, Bennett C, Paterson I, Corbishley CM, Rio MC, Chambon P and Ryall G: Expression of the pS2 gene in normal, benign and neoplastic human stomach. Int J Cancer 1989 (44):806-812
38 Wysocki S, Hahnel E, Masters A, Smith V, Mc Cartney AJ and Hahnel R: Detection of pS2 messenger RNA in gynecological cancers. Cancer Res 1990 (50):1800-1802
39 Takahashi H, Kida N, Fujii R, Tanaka K, Ohta M, Mori K and Hayashi K: Expression of the pS2 gene in human gastric cancer cells derived from poorly differentiated adenocarcinoma. FEBS Lett 1990 (261):283-286
40 Zaretsky JZ, Weiss M, Tsarfaty I, Hareuveni M, Wreschner DH and Keydar I: Expression of genes coding for pS2, c-erbB2, estrogen receptor and the H23 breast tumor associated antigen. FEBS Lett 1990 (265):46-50
41 Rio MC, Bellocq JP, Gairard B, Rasmussen UB, Krust A, Koehl C, Calderoli H, Schiff V, Renaud R and Chambon P: Specific expression of the pS2 gene in subclasses of breast cancers in comparison with expression of the estrogen and progesterone receptors and the oncogene ERBB2. Proc Natl Acad Sci USA 1987 (84):9243-9247
42 Foekens JA, Rio MC, Seguin P, Van Putten WLJ, Fauque J, Nap M, Klijn JGM and Chambon P: Prediction of relapse and survival in breast cancer patients by pS2 protein status. Cancer Res 1990 (50):3832-3837
43 Piggott NH, Henry JA, May FEB and Westley BR: Antipeptide antibodies against the pNR-2 oestrogen regulated protein of human breast cancer cells and detection of pNR-2 expression in normal tissues by immunohistochemistry.
J Pathology 1991 (163):95-104
44 Prud'homme JF, Jolivet A, Pichon MF, Savouret JF and Milgrom E: Monoclonal antibodies against native and denatured forms of estrogen induced breast cancer protein (BCEI/pS2) obtained by expression in Escherichia coli. Cancer Res 1990 (50):2390-2396
45 Schwartz LH, Koerner FC, Edgerton SM, Sawicka JM, Rio MC, Bellocq JP, Chambon P and Thor AD: pS2 expression and response to hormonal therapy in patients with advanced breast cancer. Cancer Res 1991 (51):624-628

Do All Roads Lead to the Oestrogen Receptor?

V. Craig Jordan

Department of Human Oncology, University of Wisconsin Comprehensive Cancer Center, Madison, Wisconsin 53792, U.S.A.

Beatson [1] made the initial discovery that the ovary could influence the growth of advanced breast cancer. His observation that oophorectomy could reduce the growth rate of some breast cancers was confirmed by Stanley Boyd [2] who found improvement in approximately one-third of patients. This result has been adequately supported throughout this century but it is now clear that any hormonal therapy will affect the growth rate of about one-third of advanced breast cancer in either pre- or postmenopausal women.

The reason for the apparently arbitrary response rate was discovered with the elucidation of the oestrogen receptor system in animal models [3,4] and the transfer of the technology to the clinic [5]. The determination of the steroid receptor status of a patient, to predict the hormone-responsiveness of a tumour, is now standard clinical practice in the United States. However, some have argued that the oestrogen receptor assay is redundant with the development of non-steroidal antioestrogens like tamoxifen (Nolvadex®) for the treatment of breast cancer [6]. The position can be taken that the safety of tamoxifen and its proven efficacy now mandates its use despite a negative hormone receptor result. The oestrogen receptor assay was originally introduced to reduce the numbers of oophorectomies and adrenalectomies but this is rarely a consideration today. The ubiquitous use of tamoxifen to treat selected patients at all stages of breast cancer has changed medical practice [7]. Indeed, the antioestrogens have opened up a new dimension in our strategic thinking about the oestrogen receptor system as a therapeutic target and for the development of new treatment approaches. The purpose of this chapter is to survey the current areas of research interest in hormones and their receptors and to provide the reader with an overview of the exciting possibilities for hormonal therapy in the next century.

Hormones and the Development of Breast Cancer

Oestrogen is viewed as a promoter rather than an initiator of breast cancer [8]. Women have a high incidence of breast cancer compared to men, but women with dysfunctional ovaries or who had an early oophorectomy have a low incidence of breast cancer.

During the past decade there has been considerable debate about the possibility that the early or prolonged use of oral contraceptive may increase the subsequent incidence of breast cancer. Enormous effort has been expended to detect any small changes in the breast cancer risk with the use of oral contraceptives. At present, studies either demonstrate no alteration in risk between users and non-users of oral contraceptives or slight elevations in subsequent risk.

In recent years, interest has focussed on the role of progestins in breast cancer development and growth. Intuitively, progestins have been regarded as antiproliferative agents because of their differentiating function in the uterus. This is the rationale for their use to treat endometrial carcinoma. However, it is worth pointing out that the agents used to treat endometrial carcinoma (e.g., medroxyprogesterone acetate) are not the same as the synthetic progestins found in oral contraceptives. Pike and coworkers [9] originally raised the possibility that the progestin content in oral contraceptives may be related to an increased risk of breast cancer. Recently, this view has been reinforced by Bergkvist and coworkers [10] who reported an elevated risk for breast cancer for those women who take progestins with their postmenopausal oestrogen supplements.

As a result of the aforementioned observations, we have re-examined progestins as potential promoters of breast cancer cell growth. Norethindrone is an orally active 19 nortestosterone derivative (Fig. 1). We have found [11] that norethindrone stimulates MCF-7 breast cancer cell replication and this cell growth is inhibited by antioestrogens. Indeed, norethindrone will cause all of the changes in the transforming growth factor (TGF) ß family (a group of inhibitory growth factors) normally associated with oestrogen, i.e., oestradiol and norethindrone cause a decrease in TGFß2,3 mRNA and a decrease in acid activated TGFß-like inhibitory activity in the cell culture media [11].

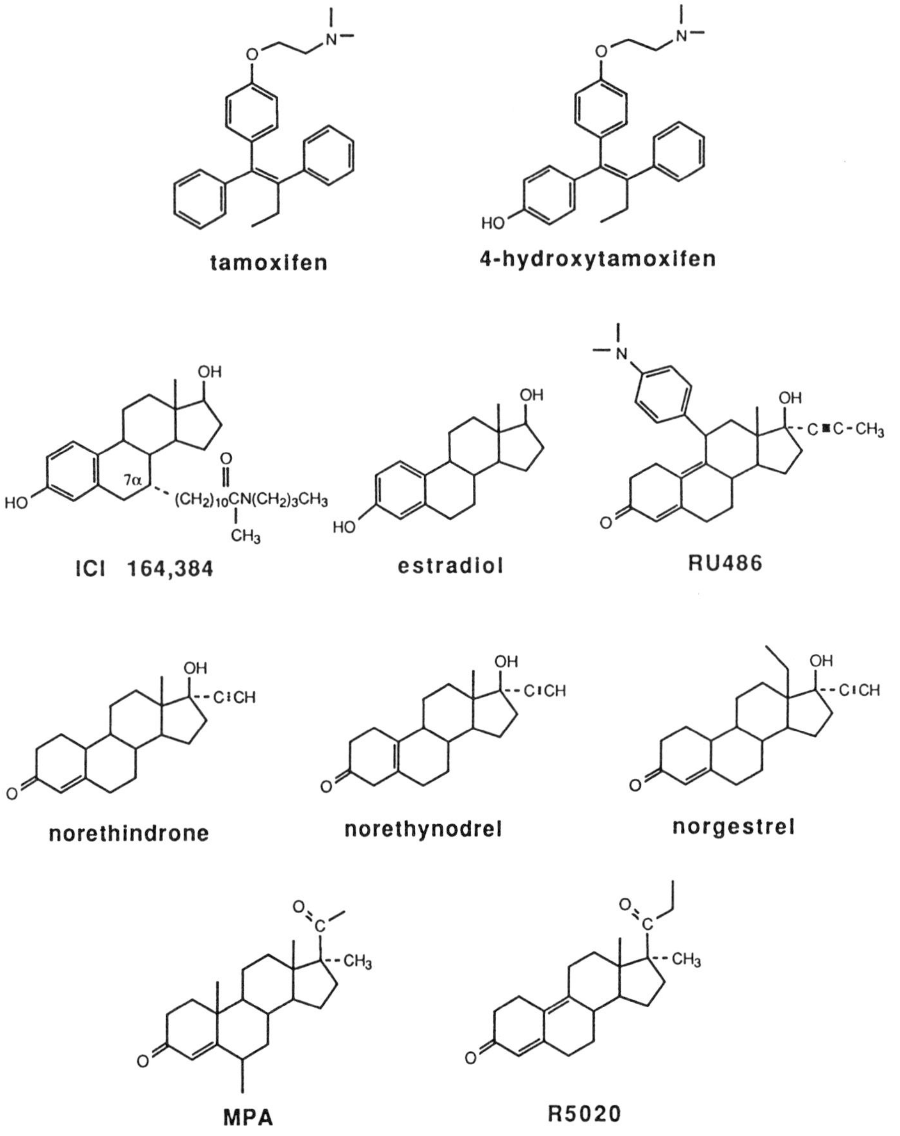

Fig. 1. The structural formulae of various hormones and antihormones mentioned in the text

Examination of other 19 nor-testosterone derivatives (norethynodrel and norgestrel) showed that each member of this family of contraceptive progestins had considerable potential to stimulate MCF-7 cell replication [12]. However, these data do not prove that progestins are functioning through the oestrogen receptor as oestrogens. Interestingly enough, though, the 19 nor-testosterone derivatives are each capable of inducing mRNA for the progesterone receptor, a marker gene for oestrogen action. Obviously, this fact demonstrates how a progestin-only contraceptive like Norplant® could work during long term (5 yrs) of treatment. Progestins cannot induce their own receptor, therefore, their action would become self limiting during weeks or months of treatment. However, if the synthetic progestin was sufficiently oestrogenic to induce progesterone receptor through an interaction with the oestrogen receptor, then indefinite action would become a reality. Proof that oestrogenic action is mediated via the oestrogen receptor can be obtained from a technique used in molecular biology. Cells can be transiently transfected with DNA constructs of reporter genes that can only be activated by specific signal mechanisms. Chloramphenicol acetyl transferase (CAT) is used as a standard reporter gene that can be activated by oestrogen receptors through an oestrogen response element (ERE) construct with a thymidine kinase promoter to regulate CAT. Only oestrogens can activate this gene through oestrogen receptors and antioestrogens will prevent the process by blocking the activation of the oestrogen receptor (Fig. 2).

All of the 19 nortestosterone derivatives will activate the CAT reporter gene transfected into MCF-7 cells and their effects can be blocked by antioestrogens [12].

Clearly, some of the progestins used in oral contraceptives could act as promoters of breast cancer growth. Epidemiological studies of *specific agents* used in oral contraceptives may reveal some important correlations with breast cancer risk. Obviously, this area needs to be evaluated very carefully before any recommendation can be made, however, the *total oestrogenicity* of preparations should be appreciated rather than maintaining the belief that low-dose progestins will be beneficial for breast cancer risk.

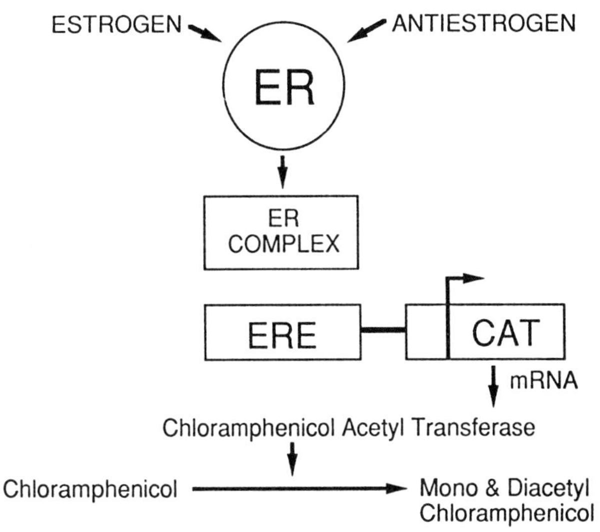

Fig. 2. Diagrammatic representation of the CAT (chloramphenicol acetyl transferase) assay with an oestrogen receptor (ER) oestrogen response element (ERE) activation system. Oestrogens can induce production of the enzyme CAT that can subsequently be assayed using radiolabelled chloramphenicol to determine the conversion to monoacetylated metabolites.

Strategy for the 1990s

Tamoxifen (Nolvadex®) is established as the endocrine treatment of choice for selected groups of patients at all stages of breast cancer [7]. Antioestrogen therapy has been so successful that there are ubiquitous applications and new approaches to treatment (Fig. 3). The successful evolution of the applications of tamoxifen to treat earlier disease has naturally resulted in the decision by the medical community to mount a controlled clinical trial in the United Kingdom to prevent breast cancer [13]. Recently, the National Cancer Institute has awarded a contract to the NSABP to develop a prevention trial with tamoxifen in America. The laboratory rationale for such a study is very strong [14-16] and an analysis of adjuvant clinical trials to determine the incidence of second primary breast cancers reveals about a 40% decrease during tamoxifen therapy [17,18]. Clearly, an evaluation of tamoxifen to prevent breast cancer is going to take up to a decade but the use of tamoxifen in women only at risk for

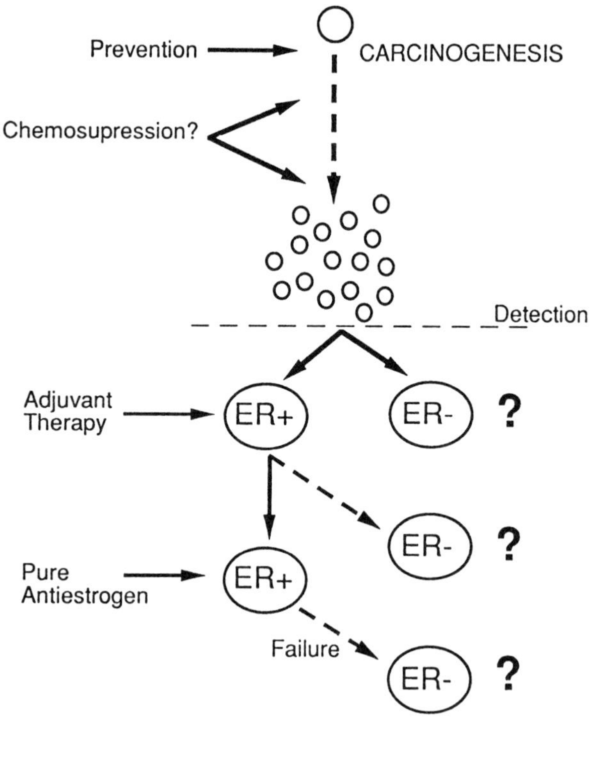

Fig. 3. Current strategies to use antioestrogens either to prevent the appearance of breast or to treat node positive or negative disease with adjuvant tamoxifen. The development of tamoxifen stimulated growth can potentially be treated with pure antioestrogens. Unfortunately, current strategies that seek to treat oestrogen receptor negative disease will probably result in only modest control.

breast cancer cannot be condoned outside a clinical trial.

The current clinical trials strategy to use adjuvant therapy is focussed on an evaluation of long-term or indefinite treatment with tamoxifen. Long-term adjuvant tamoxifen therapy (up to 5 years) is established as a safe modality to treat node-positive and negative disease that is oestrogen receptor positive. However, it is possible that the oestrogen-like properties of tamoxifen, that may prove to be so beneficial in lowering blood cholesterol [9] and maintaining bone density [20], could potentially encourage tamoxifen-stimulated breast tumour growth. We have taken the strategic step of evaluating this scenario in the laboratory. Tamoxifen will, after several years of treatment, eventually cause the growth of oestrogen receptor-positive MCF-7 breast cancer cells transplanted in athymic mice [21]. The tumours will grow with either tamoxifen or oestrogen [22] so that withdrawal of tamoxifen in the clinical situation would ultimately result in support for tumour growth from the patient's circulating oestrogen. Pure antioestrogens [23] will inhibit tamoxifen-stimulated tumour growth in the laboratory [22,24] and there are currently plans to evaluate a novel pure antioestrogen in the clinic after patients fail long-term adjuvant therapy with tamoxifen. The rapid evaluation of pure antioestrogens will place a valuable new agent in the hands of the clinician.

A Strategy for the 21st Century: "The World Turned Upside Down"

Although patients who are treated with tamoxifen for node-positive disease (and possibly node-negative disease) have a survival advantage [25], there is no evidence that patients will be cured. Regrettably, the common course of events runs from an initial responsiveness of the disease to hormonal therapy but then there is the inevitable development of receptor-negative disease that is ultimately refractory to all attempts at therapeutic control. However, the question can be asked, "If the oestrogen receptor gene was encouraged to resynthesise protein, could this transcription factor reassert cellular control?" The cDNA for the oestrogen receptor has been cloned [26] and transient transfectants have demonstrated that constitutive vectors can produce pharmacologically active protein as assessed by CAT assays.

We have taken the strategic step of constructing a novel transfection vector and developed stable transfected lines with MDA-MB-231 cloned cells. These originally receptor-negative cells are completely refractory to hormone therapy but the novel oestrogen receptor-positive transfectants are growth controlled by oestrogen. Interestingly, and unlike MCF-7 breast cancer cells whose growth is encouraged by oestradiol, the growth of the transfectants is inhibited by oestrogen. The pure antioestrogen ICI 164,384 does not affect growth but completely blocks the effect of oestrogen [27,28,].

These exciting novel data may provide the rationale for a new targeted therapy for breast cancer that is refractory to hormonal treatment. If either the oestrogen receptor gene can be reactivated selectively in these tumour cells or a way can be found to target a virus containing the cDNA for the oestrogen receptor, then perhaps a new targeted "gene therapy" may be positioned for clinical testing. Indeed, a woman's tumour may be controlled by her own postmenopausal oestrogen. In fact, we have noted that tamoxifen is sufficiently oestrogenic to be able to inhibit the growth of the transfected breast cancer cells. One could therefore imagine that tamoxifen could have a dual function to control the growth of hormone-responsive breast cancer cells and provide physiological support by lowering cholesterol and preventing bone loss. However, in addition, during the later stages of the disease tamoxifen could prevent the growth of hormone-independent breast cancer cells transfected with the new oestrogen receptor gene therapy.

In fact, the possibilities for targeted therapy with steroid receptor genes could go much further than one might at first imagine. Perhaps the oestrogen receptor can control the growth of colon cancer or lung cancer. Indeed, any cancer might now be able to be targeted for control. The possibilities might be endless and provide the clinician with a revolutionary new approach to target-site specificity. The pharmacologist has spent much effort to design drugs to activate or inactivate target tissue receptor systems. Perhaps the next generation of therapies will attempt to move the receptors to change the responses in the tissues.

Acknowledgements

I would like to thank Meei-Huey Jeng and Shun-Yuan Jiang for outstanding assistance in the laboratory to establish the scientific basis on which the proposals in this chapter are offered. Both are graduate students in the Human Cancer Biology Programme in the Department of Human Oncology at the University of Wisconsin Comprehensive Cancer Center.

REFERENCES

1 Beatson GT: On the treatment of inoperable cases of carcinoma of the mamma: Suggestions for a new method of treatment with illustrative cases. Lancet 1896 (ii):104-107

2 Boyd S: On oophorectomy in cancer of the breast. Br Med J 1920 (ii):1161-1167

3 Jensen EV, Jacobson HI: Basic guides to the mechanism of estrogen action. Recent Prog Horm Res 1962 (18):387-414

4 Toft DO, Gorski J: A receptor molecule for estrogens: Isolation from rat uterus and preliminary characterization. Proc Natl Acad Sci 1966 (55):1574-1581

5 McGuire WL, Carbone PP, Vollmer EP (eds): Estrogen Receptors in Human Breast Cancer. New York, Raven Press, 1975

6 Lerner LJ, Jordan VC: Development of antiestrogens and their use in breast cancer. Eight Cain Memorial Award Lecture. Cancer Res 1990 (50):4177-4189

7 Jordan VC, Murphy CS: Endocrine pharmacology of antiestrogens as antitumor agents. Endocr Rev 1990 (11):578-610

8 Henderson BE, Ross R, Bernstein L: Estrogens as a cause of human cancer: The Richard and Hilda Rosenthal Foundation Award lecture. Cancer Res 1988 (48):246-252

9 Pike MC, Henderson BE, Krailo MD et al: Breast cancer in young women and use of oral contraceptives: Possible modifying effects of formulation and age at first use. Lancet 1983 (i):926-930

10 Bergkvist L, Adami H-O, Persson I et al: The risk of breast cancer after estrogen and estrogen progestin replacement. N Engl J Med 1989 (321):293-297

11 Jeng MH, Jordan VC: Growth stimulation and differential regulation of TGFß1, TGFß2 and TGFß3 mRNA levels by norethindrone in MCF-7 human breast cancer cells. Mol Endocr (in press)

12 Jeng MH, Parker, CJ, Jordan VC: Estrogenic potential of progestins in oral contraceptives to stimulate human breast cancer cell proliferation. Breast Cancer Res Treat (in press)

13 Powles TJ, Tillyer CR, Jones AL et al: Prevention of breast cancer with tamoxifen - an update on the Royal Marsden Hospital pilot programme. Eur J Cancer 1990 (20):680-684

14 Jordan VC: Effect of tamoxifen (ICI 46,474) on initiation and growth of DMBA-induced rat mammary carcinomata. Eur J Cancer 1976 (12):419-423

15 Jordan VC: Chemosuppression of breast cancer with long-term tamoxifen therapy. Prev Med 1991 (20):3-14

16 Jordan VC, Lababidi MK, Langan-Fahey S: The suppression of mouse mammary tumorigenesis by long-term tamoxifen therapy. JNCI 1991 (83):492-496

17 Fisher B, Costantino J, Redmond C et al: A randomized clinical trial evaluating tamoxifen in the treatment of patients with node negative breast cancer who have estrogen receptor positive tumors. N Engl J Med 1989 (320):479-484

18 Fornander T, Rutqvist JC, Skoog L et al: Adjuvant tamoxifen in early breast cancer: occurrence of new primary cancers. Lancet 1989 (i):117-120

19 Love RR, Newcomb PA, Wiebe DA et al.: Effect of tamoxifen therapy on lipid and lipoprotein levels in postmenopausal patients with node negative breast cancer. JNCI 1990 (82):1327-1331

20 Fornander T, Rutqvist LE, Sjorberg HE et al: Long-term adjuvant tamoxifen in early breast cancer: Effect on bone mineral density in postmenopausal women. J Clin Oncol 1990 (8):1019-1026

21 Gottardis MM, Jordan VC: Development of tamoxifen-stimulated growth of MCF-7 tumors in athymic mice after long-term antiestrogen administration. Cancer Res 1988 (48):5184-5187

22 Gottardis MM, Jiang SY, Jeng MH, Jordan VC: Inhibition of tamoxifen-stimulated growth of an MCF-7 tumor variant in athymic mice by novel steroidal antiestrogens. Cancer Res 1987 (49):4090-4093

23 Wakeling AE, Bowler J: Steroidal pure antioestrogens. J Endocrinol 1987 (112):R7-R10

24 Gottardis MM, Ricchio ME, Satyaswaroop PG, Jordan VC: Effect of steroidal and non-steroidal antiestrogens on the growth of a tamoxifen-stimulated human endometrial carcinoma (En Ca 101) in athymic mice. Cancer Res 1990 (50):3189-3192

25 Early Breast Cancer Trialists' Collaborative Group: Effects of adjuvant tamoxifen and of cytotoxic therapy on mortality in early breast cancer. N Engl J Med 1988 (319):1681-1692

26 Green S, Walter P, Kumar V et al: Human oestrogen receptor cDNA; sequence expression and homology to V-erb A. Nature 1986 (320):134-139

27 Jordan VC, Jeng MH, Jiang SY, Yingling J, Stella, A: Hormonal strategies for breast cancer: A new focus on the estrogen receptor as a therapeutic target. Sem Oncol (in press)

28 Jiang SY, Jordan VC: Estrogen regulation of MDA-MB-231 breast cancer cells transfected with estrogen receptor cDNA's. Breast Cancer Res Treat (in press)

Tamoxifen for the Treatment of Breast Cancer in the Premenopausal Patient

V. Craig Jordan

Department of Human Oncology, University of Wisconsin Comprehensive Cancer Center, Madison, Wisconsin 53792, U.S.A.

Tamoxifen (Nolvadex®), a non-steroidal antioestrogen, was first introduced into clinical practice in the 1970s for the treatment of advanced breast cancer in postmenopausal patients [1-3]. Subsequent study showed that tamoxifen was also an effective palliative agent in premenopausal patients with advanced disease [4-7].

One valuable characteristic of tamoxifen therapy is the low reported incidence of side effects [8]. This, plus the proven efficacy in advanced disease, made tamoxifen an ideal agent to evaluate as an adjuvant therapy. The majority of patients entered into the early adjuvant trials of tamoxifen monotherapy were postmenopausal and early treatment schedules employed 1 or 2 years of therapy [9]. However, an overview analysis of randomised studies [9] has demonstrated a *survival* advantage for those postmenopausal women taking tamoxifen. These encouraging data have provided the incentive to apply tamoxifen more broadly. Developing laboratory [10] and clinical [11-14] evidence has indicated the value of long-term (2-5 years) adjuvant tamoxifen therapy as chemosuppressant to prevent the recurrence of node-positive disease and also the value of tamoxifen to reduce the numbers of second primary breast cancers [15-17], thus avoiding the requirement for a second mastectomy.

Several clinical studies [14,17,18] have entered premenopausal patients and these women also show benefit from adjuvant tamoxifen therapy. Indeed, the clinical alert (May 18, 1988) from the National Cancer Institute has described the value of adjuvant tamoxifen therapy for node-negative premenopausal patients who had an ER-positive primary tumour (information derived from protocol B14 from the NSABP [17]). It is possible that many hundreds of thousands of women will be taking long-term (or even indefinite) adjuvant tamoxifen therapy and an increasing proportion of these women will be premenopausal.

The aim of this chapter is to consider the pharmacological actions of tamoxifen in the premenopausal patient so that the clinician will be aware of the physiological changes and be able to evaluate possible risks.

Tamoxifen and an Alteration in Ovarian Steroidogenesis

There is some information in the literature about the impact of short-term tamoxifen administration (a few weeks to a few months) on the endocrinology of normal premenopausal women [19,20] or those with advanced breast cancer [4,7]. In general, tamoxifen causes an increase in circulating oestrogen levels and some rises in circulating progesterone. A proportion of women become amenorrhoeic during tamoxifen therapy, however, regular menstrual cycles are generally reported.

Investigators have documented the endocrinological changes that occur in premenopausal women during adjuvant chemotherapy and tamoxifen [21,22]. Young (less than 40 years old) women usually maintain ovarian function following adjuvant chemotherapy and continue to menstruate. Changes in ovarian steroidogenesis have been documented in patients maintained on long-term adjuvant tamoxifen therapy [23,24]

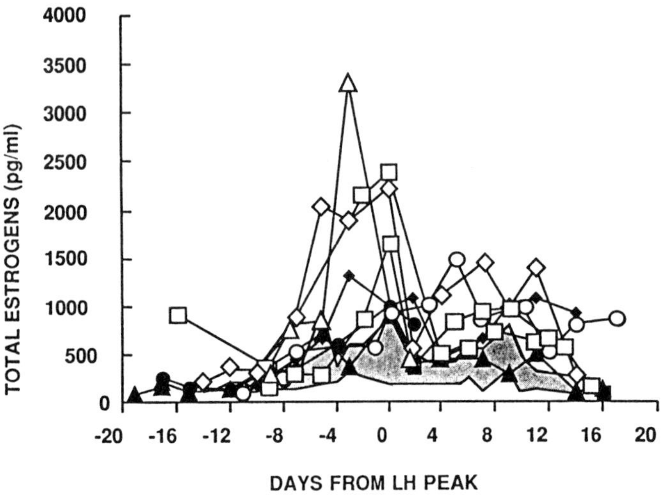

Fig. 1. The effect of adjuvant tamoxifen monotherapy (10 mg b.i.d.) on the levels of circulating total oestrogens (oestrone + oestradiol) in premenopausal patients. The range for control women is shown in the shaded area.

and in general there are increases in ovarian oestrogen production.

Clearly, it is important to appreciate the effects of tamoxifen in the premenopausal patient. In a recent study [25] we have documented the alterations in the endocrine parameters in premenopausal women with breast cancer during long-term (4-72 months) adjuvant tamoxifen monotherapy. Each of the women continued to menstruate and there were peaks of oestrogen 2-3 times the normal range (Fig. 1).

Naturally, since tamoxifen is a competitive inhibitor of oestrogen action at the oestrogen receptor it is only reasonable to consider whether the elevation in circulating oestrogen could be to the disadvantage of disease control.

Laboratory Studies with Tamoxifen

Tamoxifen inhibits the oestrogen-stimulated growth of breast cancer cells in culture [26] and at low concentrations of antioestrogen oestrogen can reverse the inhibitory action on growth. Oestrogen cannot reverse the effects of high concentrations of antioestrogens.

Similarly, tamoxifen inhibits the oestrogen-stimulated growth of tumours derived from the MCF-7 breast cancer cell line that have been inoculated into athymic mice [27,28]. We have recently determined whether increasing circulating concentrations of oestradiol can reverse the antitumour actions of tamoxifen *in vivo* and cause tumour re-growth. We used a sustained release method [29] to treat tumour-bearing athymic mice. The level of oestradiol we selected was designed to be within the range (500-900 pg/ml) normally observed in premenopausal patients during tamoxifen therapy. The sustained level of tamoxifen (40 ng/ml) was at the low end of the range normally observed in patients during long-term adjuvant therapy with tamoxifen [30] but there was a marked antitumour effect. This result is consistent with clinical experience in premenopausal patients. However, extremely high levels of oestradiol (approximately 2000 pg/ml) can reverse the action of tamoxifen and cause tumour re-growth (Fig. 2). These principles may translate directly to the clinic. Perhaps premenopausal women taking tamoxifen should be monitored to ensure they have adequate serum levels of drug in the 100-200 ng/ml range. If adequate levels of tamoxifen are present it may be unnecessary to employ methods to reduce circulating ovarian steroids. Nevertheless, concerns about the long-term effects of tamoxifen on ovarian physiology might mandate a closer evaluation in node negative patients.

Tamoxifen and Pregnancy

Tamoxifen can induce ovulation in the subfertile patient [31]. It is now clear that continuous tamoxifen therapy may not prevent ovu-

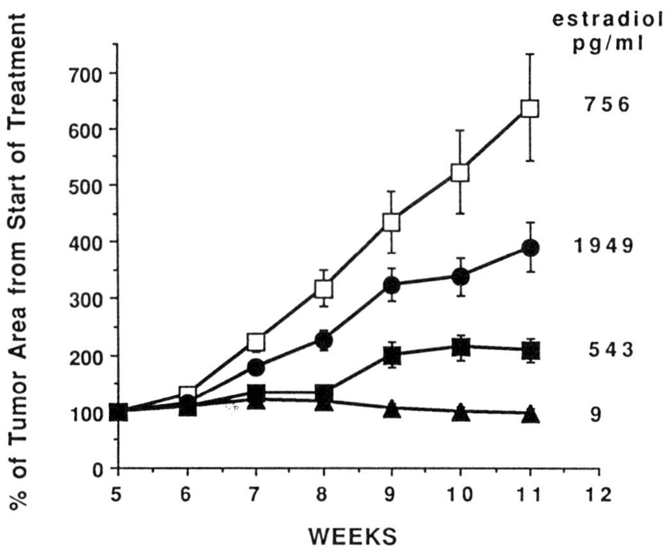

Fig. 2. Percent increase in mean tumour area plotted as mean ± SEM, or MCF-7 tumours grown in athymic mice treated with various doses of oestradiol with or without tamoxifen. The treatments are: oestradiol alone (□), tamoxifen + oestradiol high dose (●), tamoxifen + oestradiol (■), tamoxifen alone (▲). Ten mice per group.

lation so patients will remain at risk for pregnancy. There is, however, very little data about the effects of tamoxifen on the foetus primarily because most tamoxifen usage is in the postmenopausal patient. Only anecdotal experience is available in women who have taken tamoxifen inadvertently during pregnancy. Most importantly the manufacturer recommends that the drug should not be taken during pregnancy. If premenopausal patients continue to be maintained on long-term tamoxifen therapy physicians should recommend suitable methods of contraception (not, however, oral contraceptives!).
This is particularly true because some patients may be unaware of their risks of pregnancy or, in fact, that they have become pregnant. Tamoxifen therapy is associated with intermittent amenorrhoea in some premenopausal patients so a woman may not be immediately aware that she is pregnant. However, at steady state, tamoxifen has a long serum half-life (7 days) and up to 2 months may be required to clear the drug from saturated tissues [31]. It is therefore possible that the implanted and developing foetus may be exposed to tamoxifen and its metabolites throughout the critical first trimester. Although there is no evidence that tamoxifen is teratogenic in primates, the physician has a primary responsibility to advise his patients of the risks of pregnancy.

Ovarian Toxicology

Tamoxifen and the related agent clomiphene can cause ovarian enlargement [32,33] but it is not known whether tamoxifen causes deleterious effects after many years of therapy. No increase in ovarian carcinoma has been reported after long-term adjuvant tamoxifen therapy [16]. However, the patient population was postmenopausal and no assurance can be given to young premenopausal women. Clearly, future studies of the pathophysiological effects of tamoxifen on ovarian function would be prudent.

Summary

Tamoxifen is available to treat premenopausal patients with advanced breast cancer and is effective as an adjuvant therapy in both node-positive and negative disease. Long-term adjuvant therapy (2-5 years) is now commonplace in clinical practice but physicians should remain cautious and appraise patients of their risk of pregnancy. However, if patients become pregnant tamoxifen should be discontinued.
In general, tamoxifen appears to be an effective anticancer agent in the premenopausal patient despite increases in ovarian steroidogenesis. Laboratory studies indicate that oe-

strogen can reverse the effects of tamoxifen, however, adequate circulating levels of the drug (100-200 ng/ml) or a reduction in the levels of oestrogen might be expected to maintain the effectiveness of adjuvant tamoxifen therapy. Future clinical trials of tamoxifen in a reduced oestrogen environment in postmenopausal women should be undertaken to determine whether additional advantages might accrue over tamoxifen alone.

REFERENCES

1 Cole MP, Jones CTA and Todd IDH: A new antioestrogenic agent in late breast cancer. An early clinical appraisal of ICI46,474. Br J Cancer 1971 (25):270-275

2 Ward HWC: Antioestrogen therapy for breast cancer: A trial of tamoxifen at two dose levels. Br Med J 1973 (i):13-14

3 Tormey DC, Simon RM, Lippman ME et al: Evaluation of tamoxifen dose in advanced breast cancer. A progress report. Cancer Treat Rep 1976 (60):1451-1459

4 Manni A, Pearson OH: Antiestrogen-induced remissions in premenopausal women with stage IV breast cancer: Effects on ovarian function. Cancer Treat Rep 1980 (64):779-784

5 Ingle JN, Krook JE, Green ST et al: Randomized trial of bilateral oophorectomy versus tamoxifen in premenopausal women with metastatic breast cancer. J Clin Oncol 1986 (4):178-185

6 Buchanan RB, Blamey RW, Durrant KR et al: A randomized comparison of tamoxifen with surgical oophorectomy in premenopausal patients with advanced breast cancer. J Clin Oncol 1986 (4):1326-1330

7 Sawka CA, Pritchard KI, Paterson DJA et al: Role and mechanism of action of tamoxifen in premenopausal women with metastatic breast cancer. Cancer Res 1986 (46):3152-3156

8 Jordan VC, Murphy CS: Endocrine pharmacology of antiestrogens as antitumor agents. Endocr Rev 1990 (11):578-610

9 Early Breast Cancer Trialists' Collaborative Group: Effects of adjuvant tamoxifen therapy and of cytotoxic therapy on mortality in early breast cancer. N Engl J Med.1988 (319):1681-1692

10 Jordan VC: Long-term adjuvant therapy for breast cancer. In: DeVita VT, Hellman S, Rosenberg SA (eds) Important Advances in Oncology. Lippincott, Philadelphia 1984 pp 179-192

11 Tormey DC, Jordan VC: Long-term tamoxifen adjuvant therapy in node positive breast cancer: Metabolic and pilot clinical study. Breast Cancer Res Treat 1984 (4):297-302

12 Delozier T, Julien JP, Juret P et al.: Adjuvant tamoxifen in postmenopausal breast cancer: Preliminary results of a randomized trial. Breast Cancer Res Treat 1986 (7):105-110

13 Fisher B, Brown A, Wolmark N et al: Prolonging tamoxifen therapy for primary breast cancer. Ann Int Med 1987 (106):649-654

14 Breast Cancer Trials Committee, Scottish Trials Office (MRC), Edinburgh: Adjuvant tamoxifen in the management of operable breast cancer: The Scottish trial. Lancet 1987 (i):171-176

15 Cuzick J, Baum M: Tamoxifen and contralateral breast cancer. Lancet 1985 (ii):282

16 Fornander T, Rutqvist LE, Cedermark B et al: Adjuvant tamoxifen in early breast cancer: Occurrence of new primary cancers. Lancet 1989 (i):117-120

17 Fisher B, Costantino J, Redmond C et al: A randomized clinical trial evaluating tamoxifen in the treatment of patients with node negative breast cancer who have estrogen receptor-positive tumors. N Engl J Med 1985 (320):479-484

18 Cancer Research Campaign Adjuvant Trial. Cyclophosphamide and tamoxifen as adjuvant therapies in the management of breast cancer. Preliminary analysis by the CRC Adjuvant Trial Working Group. Br J Cancer 1988 (57):604-610

19 Groom GV, Griffiths K: Effects of antioestrogen tamoxifen on plasma levels of luteinizing hormone, follicle-stimulating hormone, prolactin, oestradiol, and progesterone in normal premenopausal women. J Endocrinol 1976 (70):421-428

20 Senior BVE, Cawood ML, Oakey RE et al: A comparison of the effects of clomiphene and tamoxifen treatment on the concentration of oestradiol and progesterone in the peripheral plasma of infertile women. Clin Endocrinol 1978 (8):381-389

21 Rose DP, Davis TE: Effects of adjuvant chemohormonal therapy on the ovarian and adrenal function of breast cancer patents. Cancer Res 1980 (40):4043-4047

22 Dnistrian AM, Greenberg EJ, Dillon JH et al: Chemohormonal therapy and endocrine function in breast cancer patients. Cancer 1985 (56):63-70

23 Jordan VC, Fritz NF, Tormey DC: Endocrine effects of adjuvant chemotherapy and long-term tamoxifen administration on node-positive patients with breast cancer. Cancer Res 1987 (47):624-630

24 Ravdin PM, Fritz NF, Tormey DC, Jordan VC: Endocrine status of premenopausal node-positive breast cancer patients following adjuvant chemotherapy and long term tamoxifen. Cancer Res 1988 (48):1026-1029

25 Jordan VC, Fritz NF, Langan-Fahey S, Thompson M, Tormey DC: Alteration of endocrine parameters in premenopausal women with breast cancer during long-term adjuvant tamoxifen monotherapy. JNCI (in press)

26 Lippman ME, Bolan G, Huff K: The effects of estrogen and antiestrogen on hormone responsive breast cancer in long term tissue culture. Cancer Res 1976 (36):4595-4601

27 Osborne CK, Hobbs K, Clark GM: Effect of estrogens and antiestrogens on growth of human breast cancer cells in athymic mice. JNCI 1981 5(67):584-590

28 Gottardis MM, Robinson SP, Jordan VC: Estradiol-stimulated growth of MCF-7 tumors implanted in

athymic mice: A model to study the tumoristatic action of tamoxifen. J Steroid Biochem 1988 (20):311-316
29 Robinson SP, Jordan VC: Antiestrogenic action of toremifene on hormone dependent, -independent and heterogeneous breast tumor growth in the athymic mouse. Cancer Res 1989 (49):1758-1763
30 Langan-Fahey SM, Tormey DC, Jordan VC: Tamoxifen metabolites in patients on long-term adjuvant tamoxifen therapy for breast cancer. Eur J Cancer 1990 (26):883-887
31 Furr BJA, Jordan VC: The pharmacology and clinical uses of tamoxifen. Pharm Ther 1984 (25):127-205
32 Gerhard I, Runnebaum B: Comparison between tamoxifen and clomiphene therapy in women with anovulation. Arch Gynaek 1979 (227):279-288
33 Ruiz-Velasso V, Rosas-Ameo V, Matute MM: Clinical inducers of ovulation: comparative results. Int J Fertil 1979 (24):61-64

The Multi-Drug Resistance Phenotype and its Reversal by Drugs (with Special Emphasis on Anti-Oestrogens)

S.B. Kaye

Beatson Oncology Centre, Western Infirmary, Bearsden, Glasgow G61 1BD, United Kingdom

Multi-drug resistance (MDR) is an unfortunate term, since it implies resistance to a wide range of drugs. In fact the origin of the MDR phenomenon is the preclinical observation of cross resistance to a specific group of natural products, particularly anthracyclines, vinca alkaloids and epipodophyllotoxins.

Conclusive data in a number of tumour types have shown that P-glycoprotein is an important factor in determining the presence of MDR. P-glycoprotein is a plasma membrane-associated protein whose function is to act as an energy-dependent pump. It has a molecular weight of 170 kD, with a duplicated structure and 2 drug binding sites located on the inner aspect of the cell membrane (Fig.1). In resistant cells, intracellular concentrations of cytotoxic drugs have been found to be much lower than in parallel sensitive cells, presumably through the action of P-glycoprotein [1].

However, it should also be borne in mind that certain MDR models have been described in which increased expression of P-glycoprotein is absent. Also it is important to remember that mechanisms other than P-glycoprotein-mediated MDR might underlie resistance to drugs such as adriamycin when it develops clinically. These include attenuation of topoisomerase activity, and possibly also glutathione-mediated changes in the extent of intracellular free radical damage. Nevertheless, P-glycoprotein-mediated MDR could be an important contributory factor clinically, and its relevance can be tested by examining clinical tumour material.

Initial studies concentrated on the use of cDNA probes to look for the presence of increased expression of mdr - mRNA, but recently, more informative data have come from the use of a series of monoclonal antibodies which can be used for immunohistochemical examination of tumour material. Valuable information on P-glycoprotein expression according to cell type can be obtained in this way [2].

P-Glycoprotein Expression in Breast Cancer

It has now been established that P-glycoprotein is encoded by a family of 3 genes in rodents (mdr 1,2 and 3) and by 2 genes in humans (mdr 1 and 3). Previous experimental data have indicated that the products of mdr 1 and 2 genes (the classes I and II isoforms of P-glycoprotein) were those primarily involved in MDR, but recent circumstantial data from resistant leukaemia cells suggest that the class 3 isoform may also have a role, although its exact function remains unclear [2].

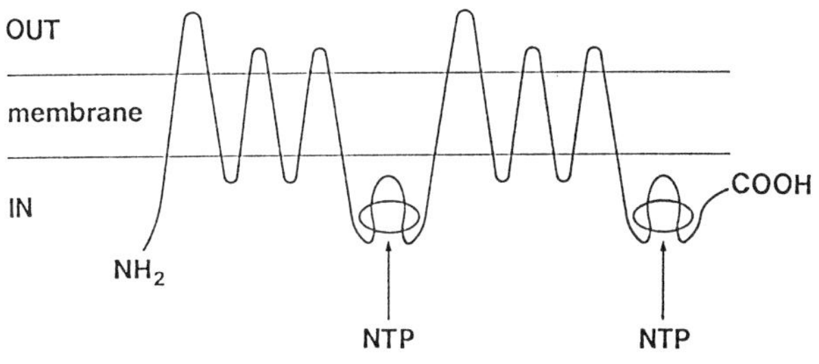

Fig. 1. Model of P-glycoprotein, showing 12 transmembrane regions and 2 intracytoplasmic nucleotide-binding sites

Table 1. Immunohistochemical detection of P-glycoprotein in breast cancer

Antibody	No.*/No. pos./tested	Clinical history	Author
MRK16	1/9	untreated	Sugarawa [9]
C219	10/23	12 (2 pos) untreated 11 (8 pos) pre-treated	Schneider [10]
MRK16 and C219	21/29	untreated	Wishart [6]
C219	20/40	pre-treated	Ro [7]
JSB-1, MRK16 and C219	3/6	unknown	Van der Valk [8]
C494	17/20	untreated	Verrelle [11]

* level of positivity varies from few to many cells

Knowledge of the existence of several isoforms of P-glycoprotein is important in assessing the available information on immunohistochemical detection of P-glycoprotein in breast cancer, since a number of studies have been published using a range of monoclonal antibodies. These antibodies have varying specificities, and this is summarised in Table 1.

Prior to the application of these monoclonal antibodies, the initial reports examining breast cancer material for increased mdr expression suggested that this would be an unlikely event. These studies used cDNA probes, and levels of mdr 1 - mRNA were compared with those present in mdr-positive breast cancer cell lines. Goldstein et al. [3] found detectable levels of mdr 1 - mRNA in only 9 of 57 untreated breast cancer biopsies, while Merkel et al. [4] found no mdr 1 - mRNA in 53 biopsies. This technique suffers, however, from the potential inability to detect a small number of positive cells in a large proportion of normal cells. Nevertheless, using these methods in a study in Glasgow, Keith et al. [5] were able to detect increased levels of mdr 1 - mRNA in approximately 50% of a series of cases of untreated breast cancer and the differences may relate to technical variations in hybridisation conditions. Of note was the fact that the range of increased expression was extremely high (up to 100) and this confirmed our view that immunohistochemical data should provide more useful information on cell type.

Of the immunohistochemical studies published to date, the majority have indicated that increased expression of P-glycoprotein is a relatively common event. In addition, positive staining of certain normal cells within breast tumours has been seen, both in stroma and in epithelial cells lining normal ducts [6,7]. Confirmatory data on P-glycoprotein staining in glandular epithelium in normal breasts have been provided by a separate study [8]. This raises the issue of the normal physiological role of P-glycoprotein (which is also present in high concentrations in other normal organs such as the adrenal gland and within the hepato-biliary system), and the potential problems which might arise as a result of attempts to inhibit its function. This will be considered further under "clinical studies".

The initial immunohistochemical studies which examined breast cancer biopsies both used a single monoclonal antibody. Sugawara et al. [9] used the MRK16 antibody and found one positive in 9 samples, while Schneider et al. [10] used the C219 antibody and found 10 positives in 23 samples with an apparently higher rate of positivity in samples from patients previously treated with "MDR" drugs. However, there are limitations to the interpretation of single antibody studies. For C219, cross-reactivity with a certain type of myosin in striated muscle has been reported, and the possibility that MRK16 may cross-react with molecules other than P-glycoprotein has been raised by Van der Valk and coworkers [8].

For these reasons, the Dutch group recommended the use of a small panel of anti-P-glycoprotein antibodies. Wishart and co-workers [6] did use 2 antibodies (C219 and MRK16) in 29 samples and demonstrated P-glycoprotein expression in epithelial cells in 21 and 16 cases, respectively. In this, and in other studies, the proportion of tumour cells which stained positive varied. In the majority of cases, positive staining was seen in up to 10% of tumour cells, while in a minority of samples up to 50% of tumour cells were positive for P-gyp. Similar observations were made for the positively-staining normal stromal cells, which were seen to a varying extent in the majority of cases.

A preliminary follow-up of the patients in the study of Wishart et al. [6] suggested a shorter disease-free survival for those patients with a higher proportion of P-gyp.-positive cells, but the numbers at present are too small to reach statistical significance [Wishart, personal communication].

In the report from Verrelle et al. [11], significant clinical correlations were identified. This study dealt with 20 patients (17 with locally advanced disease) and the C494 antibody was used to detect P-gyp in a total of 17 samples. This antibody does at present appear to be the most specific for an internal epitope (different to that for C219) on the class I isoform of P-glycoprotein. An attempt to express the results semi-quantitatively was made, taking account of both the number of positive tumour cells and the intensity of staining. Patients were treated with adriamycin-containing chemotherapy schedules, and the outcome of treatment (progression-free survival) was compared with P-gyp. expression. Interestingly, a significant correlation existed, with the most strongly positive cases exhibiting the shortest progression-free survival ($p < 0.02$). However, and as Dalton and Grogan [12] have pointed out, the number of patients in this study is small, and the impact of other potentially important prognostic factors has not been taken into account.

Nevertheless, support for the hypothesis that P-gyp. positivity does relate to chemo-resistance comes from the study by Ro et al. [7]. In their study, analysis was conducted, using the C219 antibody alone, on 48 samples, 40 of which were mastectomy samples taken after 3 cycles of adriamycin-containing chemotherapy. P-gyp. expression was seen in 20 tumours (ranging from less than 5% to 30% of tumour cells), and a significant correlation ($p = 0.005$) was seen between clinical response and the presence of P-gyp. positive tumour cells.

At present, therefore, intriguing observations have been made in respect of P-gyp. positivity and breast cancer, and the task now is to clarify its clinical relevance. Reliable immunohistochemical techniques which may be applied to formalin-fixed material would be extremely useful in this respect, in order to permit correlations with outcome in large numbers of cases.

Experimental Modulation of MDR in Breast Cancer

Verapamil was first chosen by Tsuruo as a modulator for resistance to natural products, as calcium flux was considered then to be a possible factor[13]. Subsequently, the role of P-glycoprotein was established, and calcium flux has been shown not to be important. Also a range of compounds other than verapamil have been tested. It is now clear from studies using photo-active analogues, that many of these compounds are capable of binding specifically to P-glycoprotein (although the differing specificity of the 2 binding sites in P-glycoprotein is currently being clarified) [14]. Through this action, intracellular concentrations of agents such as the anthracyclines can be increased in experimental models of MDR, and in several cases a dose-response relationship for this effect has been established for the modulating agent.

Other mechanisms for this effect, however, probably operate. For example, certain drugs are known to change membrane fluidity, and thereby will alter the characteristics of drug influx and efflux. Examples include perhexiline, and it is thought likely that the anti-oestrogen, tamoxifen, may also have this effect. An additional mechanism which may relate to tamoxifen is inhibition of the action of the protein kinase C family of enzymes. The extent of phosphorylation of P-glycoprotein may affect its function. Protein kinase C antagonists may inhibit P-glycoprotein function by reducing the degree of phosphorylation, although the data in support of this are indirect.

Tamoxifen was first identified as an MDR modulator in 1984 in experiments using P388 leukaemia cells [15]. In that study, a concentration of 6 µmol was necessary to achieve reversal of resistance *in vitro*, and transport studies using ^{3}H-labelled adriamycin confirmed that the effect of tamoxifen was to increase intracellular drug concentrations in resistant cells. Furthermore, this effect was not blocked by coincubation with 17 beta-oestradiol. Foster et al. confirmed that tamoxifen could exert this effect in mdr-positive human breast cancer cells *in vitro* [16].

A number of clinical trials using high dose tamoxifen have now confirmed that concentrations approaching those which are active *in vitro* may be achieved in plasma, although side effects (chiefly neurological) may occur (see below).

More recently, the new triphenylethylene compound, toremifene, has been noted to possess similar activity in terms of MDR modulation *in vitro* [17]. De Gregorio and co-workers, again using adriamycin-resistant human breast cancer cells *in vitro*, examined the modulating activity of toremifene and several of its metabolites. They also examined the modulating activity of an ultrafiltrate of plasma containing unbound toremifene, taken from patients who had been given toremifene at doses of 20-400 mg per day as part of a clinical study. Comparisons were also made with tamoxifen in the same report. Its main conclusions were that toremifene and its major metabolite, N-desmethyl toremifene, were capable of sensitising resistant cells at similar concentrations *in vitro* and the effective range of concentration, 2.5-10 µmol, was similar to that for tamoxifen, with a similar magnitude of effect. Encouragingly, this effect was also seen to some extent using the plasma ultra-filtrates, at least in those taken from patients given the highest dose (400 mg daily).

In attempting to correlate *in vitro* data with information on clinically achievable concentrations of modulating agents, it is necessary to consider both the extent of plasma protein binding, and perhaps more importantly the concentration of modulating agents in the tumour itself. Many of the agents concerned are extensively protein bound, and Chaterjee and Harris [18] have pointed out with respect to toremifene, that binding to alpha 1 acid glycoprotein should also be considered. Interestingly, their study, albeit with a different tumour model (Chinese Hamster ovary cells), showed that although toremifene modulated the activity of adriamycin at concentrations of 5-10 µmol, this effect was also seen in the sensitive counterpart. Moreover, no apparent change in intracellular concentration of adriamycin was found, raising the possibility of an alternative mechanism of action for toremifene, perhaps independent of P-glycoprotein.

In their study, the addition of exogenous alpha 1 acid glycoprotein almost completely abrogated the modulating effect of toremifene, and they sounded a note of caution in this respect, particularly as it is known that cancer patients may have particularly high levels of circulating alpha 1 acid glycoprotein.

However, other groups have concentrated on measurements of modulating agent levels in tumour biopsies, with interesting preliminary results. For example Wishart et al. [19] measured quinidine concentrations in tumour biopsies from a small number of breast cancer patients who had received 5 days of oral quinidine as part of a pilot trial (to be described below). Concentrations in the samples measured were comparable to those in the plasma (1-2 µmol).

For tamoxifen, studies with human tumour xenografts indicate that tumour concentrations may in fact exceed those present in the plasma by up to 100-fold. Preliminary data on tamoxifen concentrations in tumour biopsies from patients given high-dose tamoxifen are similarly encouraging [Jordan, personal communication]. Further detailed studies are therefore warranted; in particular it would be important to develop the methodology to assess concentrations of unbound modulating agents in tumour cells themselves, since those tumour concentrations noted presumably could still reflect mainly protein-bound drug in extracellular fluid.

Clinical Studies

Initial clinical studies using putative MDR modulators concentrated on the use of verapamil. Some preliminary encouraging data were reported by Presant et al. [20], but patient numbers were very small. It was soon pointed out in a pilot study in ovarian cancer by Ozols et al. [21] using verapamil by infusion in conjunction with adriamycin that attempts to reach plasma concentrations in the effective *in vitro* range (over 6 μm) were likely to be unsuccessful because of cardiotoxicity.
A further problem with the use of verapamil, discussed by Kerr et al. [22], is the possibility of pharmacokinetic interactions between this drug and cytotoxic agents such as adriamycin, by virtue of its effect on hepatic and possibly renal blood flow.
Nevertheless, verapamil has remained the lead compound in clinical trials, and despite these reservations it has been used with encouraging preliminary results in patients with refractory multiple myeloma and non-Hodgkin's lymphoma [23]. Although numbers of cases are small and studies to date have been non-randomised, clinical responses have been noted in cases with proven P-gyp-positive tumours with the use of "MDR" drugs in conjunction with verapamil infusions.
Verapamil is a racemic mixture of D and L-isomers, and the D-isomer possesses somewhat lower levels of cardioactivity but comparable levels of MDR-modulating efficacy compared to the racemic mixture [24]. Clinical trials of D-verapamil have therefore been conducted, and in the first study it appears that a modest advantage over the racemic mixture can be obtained, although the concentrations achievable may still fall somewhat short of the optimal [25]. Data from other trials are awaited. On the positive side, it is also known that the major metabolite of the racemic mixture and its isomers is nor-verapamil, and this in fact is present in equimolar concentrations after oral administration and has equivalent modulating capacity *in vitro* [26].
However, attention has increasingly turned to alternative modulating agents. In all cases these had been synthesised for the management of other conditions, ranging from cardiovascular disorders to fungal infections, and from depressive illness to post-transplant immunosuppression. For this reason, and with increasing appreciation of the structure-activity relationships of MDR-modulating agents [27], compounds specifically synthesised for this purpose are now being developed.
As has been mentioned previously, correlations between achievable plasma levels and effective *in vitro* concentrations should be interpreted with care, but they have guided selections of agents to a considerable extent, and data on a number of compounds are summarised in Table 2.
As regards those compounds initially developed for cardiovascular disease, quinidine is perhaps the most promising, particularly in respect of breast cancer. At concentrations similar to those used for verapamil, quinidine is an effective modulating agent for MCF7 adriamycin-resistant breast cancer cells *in vitro* [28]. We have also shown activity for quinidine *in vivo* in preliminary studies using xenografts of (ovarian) P-gyp.-positive human tumours [Plumb et al., personal communication].
A pilot study in patients with breast cancer receiving single-agent epirubicin confirmed the feasibility of using quinidine as an MDR modulator. Doses of 250 mg. b.d., given for 4 days prior to chemotherapy, led to plasma concentrations of approximately 6 μm, in the absence of any significant toxicity [29].

Table 2. Correlation between *in vitro* and plasma concentrations for MDR modulators

Modulator	Optimal *in vitro* concentration	Clinically achievable plasma concentration
Verapamil	6 μM	1 - 2 μM
D-verapamil	6 μM	?
Quinidine	6 μM	6 μM
Amiodarone	2 μM	2 - 6 μM
Bepridil	6 μM	2 - 4 μM
RO 11-2903 (DMDP)	1 - 4 μM	?
Trifluoperazine	1 - 6 μg/ml	130 ng/ml
Trans-flupenthixol	8 μM	?
Cyclosporin-A	1 - 5 μg/ml	1 - 6 μg/ml
Cefoperazone	1 mM	up to 1 mM
Tamoxifen	2 - 6 μM	up to 6 μM
Toremifene	2.5 - 5 μM	3 - 6 μM

With respect to the antioestrogens, two clinical trials using high-dose tamoxifen as an MDR modulator have been reported. Cantwell et al. [30] used tamoxifen in doses of 120 to 480 mg/day for up to 6 days, in conjunction with oral etoposide (300 mg daily for 3 days). Neurological side-effects and vomiting were seen at the highest dose levels. Plasma concentrations of tamoxifen of 3 to 4 μm were measured in patients receiving 320 mg per day.

Trump et al. [31] completed a phase I trial in which patients received oral tamoxifen for 13 days at doses of 40 to 260 mg/m^2 twice daily. This was given with a 5-day infusion of vinblastine (1.5 mg/m^2/day). Neurotoxicity was dose-limiting for tamoxifen; it was manifest by tremor and gait disturbances and was first noted at doses above 150 mg/m^2 b.d. Mean plasma concentrations of tamoxifen and n-desmethyl-tamoxifen (which is also an effective modulator) were 3.2 and 4.3 μm at the dose of 150 mg/m^2 b.d., and were 6.1 and 6.6 μm, respectively, at the highest dose of 260 mg/m^2 b.d. The authors concluded that effective concentrations could be reached safely, without major toxicity, at the dose of tamoxifen of 150 mg/m^2 b.d. for 13 days.

To date, in the pilot trials using tamoxifen as an MDR modulator there has been no evidence of increased toxicity, nor of obviously enhanced antitumour efficacy, although isolated responses in patients with gastric and ovarian cancer, sarcoma, and melanoma were seen in the study of the Newcastle group [30]. Tamoxifen has also been used clinically in combination with verapamil despite the absence of convincing laboratory data for either an additive or synergistic effect. At any rate, these agents have non-overlapping normal tissue toxicity, and for this reason, and taking an empirical approach, Figueredo et al. [32] performed a non-randomised trial in small cell lung cancer in which patients received chemotherapy (including adriamycin and etoposide) together with tamoxifen and verapamil. They proposed that the response rate and survival seen was superior to that seen in previous studies, but in the absence of randomised trials, such data are difficult to assess, particularly in small cell lung cancer.

With regard to toremifene, in the study of De Gregorio et al. [17] 4 patients received 200 mg daily and 9 received 400 mg daily. Vertigo and nausea are dose-limiting for high-dose toremifene, and other studies have indicated that the dose of 200 mg daily is generally well tolerated. The mean plasma concentrations of toremifene and N-desmethyl toremifene (an equally effective modulator *in vitro*) were 2.35 and 9.9 μm at the dose of 200 mg daily, and 5.75 and 19.8 μm at the dose of 400 mg daily. These concentrations, as described previously, are clearly within an effective range, notwithstanding earlier comments on protein-binding and tumour concentrations.

Another agent which has received considerable attention is cyclosporin, because of its high level of efficacy *in vitro* and the likelihood of achieving therapeutic concentrations clinically [33]. A number of schedules have been tested and the concentrations achieved have been considered appropriate [34,35]. However, the agent is primarily an immunosuppressive drug, and analogues without this activity, but retaining MDR modulating efficacy, are currently under development [36].

To date, these pilot trials have demonstrated the feasibility of the approach, but, with the exception of the data in myeloma and non-Hodgkin's lymphoma, no evidence of enhanced activity in tumours such as renal or colon cancer has yet been seen. In general terms, evidence of effective modulation through the MDR mechanism clinically may be obtained in 2 ways; either in non-randomised studies of previously refractory tumours such as renal cancer, or in randomised trials in initially sensitive tumours where resistant cells expressing P-glycoprotein may emerge following treatment. Possible examples of this, as described previously, include breast cancer as well as haematological malignancies such as acute myeloid leukaemia. A logical trial design in these cases would involve randomisation to initial treatment with an "MDR" drug with/without a modulating agent, with response rate and disease-free survival as end-points. We are currently conducting this type of (placebo controlled) randomised trial in patients with advanced breast cancer, treated with single-agent epirubicin, with/without a 5 day course of oral quinidine. A minimum of 200 patients are required, in order to detect a 50% improvement in response rate, e.g., from 40% to 60%, and

clearly the extent of any improvement could be significantly smaller.
The factors bearing on the likelihood of benefit include :

a) achievement of an effective modulating agent concentration at the tumour cell (as described above).

b) the proportion of P-gyp.-positive cells present at the stage of attempted modulation.

c) existence of multiple cellular mechanisms underlying drug resistance clinically.

Clearly it is very likely that several mechanisms including P-glycoprotein-mediated MDR will indeed co-exist. For adriamycin-resistance in breast cancer, for example, defective topoisomerase II activity may well be an important factor.
As the tools for examining these various mechanisms continue to be developed it is important to continue to examine clinical material for basic information on relevant factors, while continuing to explore the clinical potential of those modulating agents which have already been identified.

Summary

A major obstacle to improvement in the treatment of breast cancer is the development of resistance to chemotherapy, particularly adriamycin. In recent years, the role of P-glycoprotein in so-called "multi-drug resistance" to certain drugs has been elucidated. Using a variety of techniques, clinical material can now be examined for the presence of P-glycoprotein.
Data in breast cancer indicate that P-glycoprotein-positive tumour cells are present to a varying extent in a substantial number of cases. Preliminary attempts to correlate this with treatment outcome are encouraging.
The possibility should be borne in mind, however, that P-glycoprotein positivity could represent an adverse biological characteristic, not directly related to drug resistance.
If P-glycoprotein-mediated resistance to adriamycin were to be an important factor in breast cancer, its importance lies in the potential for reversal with membrane active non-cytotoxic agents. In adriamycin-resistant breast cancer cells *in vitro*, a range of agents have been found to be effective in this context. These include the anti-oestrogens, tamoxifen and toremifene, as well as the cardio-active drugs, verapamil and quinidine. The ability to achieve adequate concentrations clinically could be a limiting factor, and to that extent agents such as toremifene and quinidine are attractive candidates. Appropriate randomised clinical trials are now under way.

REFERENCES

1 Bradley G, Jwanka PF and Ling V: Mechanism of multidrug resistance. Biochem Biophys Acta 1988 (948):87-88
2 Nooter K and Herweijer H: Multidrug resistance genes in human cancer. Br J Cancer 1991 (63):663-669
3 Goldstein LJ, Galski H, Fojo A et al: Expression of a multi-drug resistance gene in human cancers. JNCI 1989 (81):116-124X
4 Merkel DE, Fuqua SA, Tandon AK, Hill SM, Buzdar AV and McGuire WL: Electrophoretic analysis of 248 clinical breast cancer specimens for P glycoprotein overexpression or gene amplification. J Clin Oncol 1989 (7):1129-1136
5 Keith WN, Stallard S and Brown R: Expression of mdr-1 and gst-pi in human breast tumours: comparison to in vitro chemosensitivity. Br J Cancer 1990 (61):712-716
6 Wishart GC, Plumb JA, Goring JJ, McNicol AM, McArdle CS, Tsuruo T, and Kaye SB: P-glycoprotein expression in primary breast cancer detected by immunocytochemistry with 2 monoclonal antibodies. Br J Cancer 1990 (62):758-761
7 Ro J, Sahin A, Ro JY, Fritsche H, Hortobagyl G and Blick M: Immunohistochemical analysis of P-glycoprotein expression correlated with chemotherapy resistance in locally advanced breast cancer. Hum Pathol 1990 (21):787-791
8 Van der Valk P, Van Kalken C, Ketslaars H, Broxterman HJ, Scheffer G, Kniper C, Tsuruo T, Lankelma J, Meijer CJ, Pinedo HM and Scheper RJ: Distribution of multi-drug resistance-associated P-glycoprotein in normal and neoplastic human tissues. Ann Oncol 1990 (1):56-64
9 Sugawara I, Kataoka I, Morishita Y et al: Tissue distribution of P-glycoprotein encoded by a multidrug resistant gene as revealed by a monoclonal antibody, MRK-16. Cancer Res 1988 (48):1926-1929
10 Schneider J, Bak M, Efferth T, Kaufmann M, Mattern J, and Volm M: P-glycoprotein expression in treated and untreated human breast cancer. Br J Cancer 1989 (60):815-818
11 Verrelle P, Meissonnier F, Fonck Y, Feillel V, Dionet C, Kwiatkowski F, Plague R, and Chassagne J: Clinical relevance of immunohistochemical detection of multidrug resistance P-glycoprotein in breast carcinoma. JNCI 1991 (83):111-116
12 Dalton W and Grogan TM: Does P-glycoprotein predict response to chemotherapy, and if so, is there a reliable way to detect it. JNCI 1991 (83):80-82
13 Tsuruo T, Lida H, Tsukagoslin S, Sakwai Y: Overcoming of vincristine resistance in P388 leukaemia through enhanced cytotoxicity by verapamil. Cancer Res 1981 (41) 1967-1972
14 Safa AR: Photoaffinity labelling of P-glycoprotein with photoactive analogues of verapamil. Proc Natl Acad Sci 1988 (85):7187 - 7190
15 Ramu A, Glaubiger D and Fuks Z: Reversal of acquired resistance to doxorubicin in P388 cells by tamoxifen and other triparamol analogues. Cancer Res 1984 (44):4392-4396
16 Foster BJ, Grotzinger KR, McKay M et al: Modulation of induced resistance to adriamycin in two human breast cancer cell lines with tamoxifen or perhexilene maleate. Cancer Chemother Pharmacol 1988 (22):147-152
17 DeGregorio MW, Ford JM, Benz CC, Wiebe VJ: Toremifene: Pharmacologic and pharmacokinetic basis of reversing multidrug resistance. J Clin Oncol 1989 (7):1359-1364
18 Chatterjee M and Harris AL: Enhancement of adriamycin cytotoxicity in a multidrug resistant Chinese Hamster Ovary (CHO) Subline, CHO-Adr, by toremifene and its modulation by alpha, acid glycoprotein. Eur J Cancer 1990 (26):432-436
19 Wishart GC, Morrison JG, Plumb JA et al: In a randomized trial in breast cancer, quinidine does not increase epirubicin toxicity, but adequate tumour levels can be detected. Proc Amer Soc Clin Oncol 1991 (10):52
20 Presant CA, Kennedy PS, Wiseman C et al: Verapamil reversal of clinical doxorubicin resistance in human cancer. Am J Clin Oncol 1986 (9):355-357
21 Ozols RF, Cynnion RE, Klecker RW et al: Verapamil and adriamycin in the treatment of drug-resistant ovarian cancer patients. J Clin Oncol 1987 (5):641-647
22 Kerr DJ, Graham J, Cummings J et al: The effect of verapamil on the pharmacokinetics of adriamycin. Cancer Chemother Pharmacol 1986 (18):239-242
23 Dalton WS, Grogan TM, Meltzer PS et al: Drug-resistance in multiple myeloma and non Hodgkin's lymphoma: detection of P glycoprotein and potential circumvention with verapamil. J Clin Oncol1989 (7):415-417
24 Plumb JA, Milroy R and Kaye SB: The activity of verapamil as a resistance modifier in vitro in drug resistant human tumour cell lines is not stereospecific. Biochem Pharmacol 1990 (39):787-792
25 Bissett D, Kerr DJ, Cassidy J, Meredith P and Kaye SB: Phase I study of D-verapamil and doxorubicin. Ann Oncol 1990 (Supp 1):117
26 Merry S, Flanigan P, Schlick E, Freshney RI and Kaye SB: Inherent adriamycin resistance in a rodent tumour line: circumvention with verapamil and norverapamil. Br J Cancer 1989 (59):895-897
27 Pearce HL, Safa AR, Back NJ, Winter MA, Cirtain MC and Beck WT: Essential features of the P glycoprotein pharmacophore. Proc Natl Acad Sci USA 1989 (86):5128-5130
28 Plumb JA: Modulation of drug resistance in vitro and in vivo. Anticancer Res 1990 (10):1401
29 Jones RD, Kerr DJ, Harnett AN, Rankin EM, Ray S and Kaye SB: A pilot study of quinidine and epirubicin in the treatment of advanced breast cancer. Br J Cancer 1990 (62):133-135
30 Cantwell B, Carmichael J, Millward M, Chatterjee M and Harris AL: Intermittent high dose tamoxifen with oral etopside - Phase I + II clinical studies. Proc Am Soc Clin Oncol 1989 (8):65
31 Trump DL, Smith DC, Schold SC, Rogers MP, Ellis PG, Fine RL, Winer EP, Pinella TJ and Jordan VC: High dose tamoxifen and 5-day continuous infusion

vinblastine: A phase I trial of an inhibitor of the MDR-1 phenotype. Proc Am Soc Clin Oncol 1991 (10):96
32 Figueredo A, Arnold A, Goodyear M et al: Addition of verapamil and tamoxifen to the initial chemotherapy of small cell lung cancer. Cancer 1990 (65):1895-1899
33 Slater LM, Sweet, Stupecky M and Gupta S: Cyclosporin A reverses vincristine and daumorubicin resistance in acute lymphatic leukaemia in vitro. J Clin Invest 1986 (77):1405-1408
34 Verweij J, Herweijer H, Planting A, Rodenburg C, Boersma G, Stoter G and Nooter K: In vitro and in vivo studies on the efficacy of cyclosporin A in the circumvention of clinical multidrug resistance. Proc Am Soc Clin Oncol 1990 (9):74
35 Yahanda AM, Adler KM, Hardy R, Brophy NA, Halsey J and Sikic BI: A phase I trial of etoposide with cyclosporin as a modulator of multidrug resistance. Proc Am Soc Clin Oncol 1991 (10):102
36 Twentyman PR: Modification of cytotoxic drug resistance by non-immunosuppressive cyclosporins. Br J Cancer 1988 (57):254

New Endocrine Agents for Breast Cancer

Andrea Manni

Division of Endocrinology, Department of Medicine, The Pennsylvania State University, The Milton S. Hershey Medical Center, Hershey, PA 17033, U.S.A.

The treatment of breast cancer still requires considerable improvement. The introduction of modern endocrine agents such as antioestrogens and aromatase inhibitors has substantially reduced the toxicity associated with major ablative surgical procedures such as adrenalectomy and hypophysectomy and consequently has enhanced the practical applicability of hormone therapy [1]. However, response rate, duration of response and survival in patients with metastatic disease have not been improved [1]. Likewise, the palliative effects of chemotherapy have remained essentially unchanged since the early 70s when adriamycin containing combination regimens were first introduced [2]. In addition, the beneficial effects of endocrine therapy and chemotherapy in patients with early disease, although encouraging, remain restricted to a relatively small fraction of women [1].

It is obvious that in order to develop improved treatment strategies, it is necessary to have a deeper understanding of the basic mechanisms which control breast cancer cell proliferation. Recent evidence suggests an important role for autocrine/paracrine factors in the control of tumour growth. A schematic representation of such basic mechanisms is illustrated in Figure 1. An increasing number of polypeptide growth factors have been found to be produced by breast cancer cells and in hormone-dependent human breast cancer cell lines their secretion has been shown to be hormonally regulated [3-6]. In addition, breast cancer cells possess receptors for such growth factors and manifest a significant proliferative response when exposed to these peptides [3,7-9]. Stromal-epithelial interactions probably play an important role in the autocrine/paracrine control of breast cancer growth. For instance, certain growth factors such as insulin-like growth factor-I (IGF-I) appear to be produced by stromal cells but may

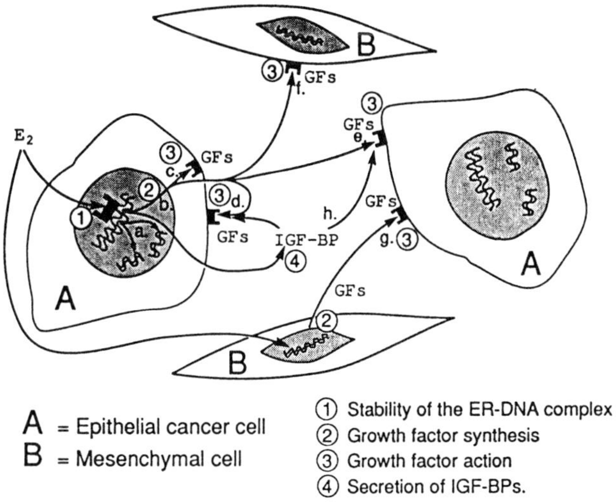

Fig. 1. Potential steps in the hormonal control of breast cancer cell proliferation affected by polyamines. Following association with E_2, the oestrogen receptor binds to specific DNA acceptor sites where it initiates transcription. E_2 promotes breast cancer cell proliferation either directly through stimulation of DNA replicating enzymes (a) or indirectly through induction of growth factor (GF) production (b). Such GFs act on the cell of origin through an intracrine (c) or an autocrine (d) mechanism (depending on whether or not they are secreted into the extracellular space). They also stimulate proliferation of neighbouring cells (paracrine effect) either epithelial (e) or mesenchymal (f). Some GFs (i.e., IGF-I) are produced by mesenchymal cells and stimulate the growth of epithelial cancer cells (g). Insulin-like growth factor binding proteins (IGF-BP) also may play an important role in modulating IGF action. Circled numbers indicate the steps in this complex control of growth potentiality influenced by polyamines.

be exerting a mitogenic effect on the surrounding epithelial cells [10]. The reverse situation is probably true for other growth factors such as platelet-derived growth factor (PDGF) [11]. With regard to the roles of IGF-I and -II, an additional level of complexity has been introduced by the recent discovery that breast cancer cells also secrete a large number of IGF-binding proteins [12-14] which may, in turn, significantly modulate the effects of IGFs on tumour cell proliferation [15,16].

Over the last several years, our laboratory has been interested in studying the role of polyamines (putrescine, spermidine and spermine) in breast cancer growth with specific emphasis on the interactions between the polyamine and autocrine/paracrine pathways. Figure 1 illustrates the potential specific sites of interplay between hormones and polyamines in the control of breast cancer growth. A possible interaction is at the hormone receptor level since polyamines have been shown to affect the structure and stability of the oestrogen receptor complex [17]. In addition, they have also been found to be capable of enhancing the binding of progesterone receptor to DNA [18]. Data from our own laboratory have suggested an important role of polyamines in growth factor action [19-22] and, under selected circumstances, growth factor synthesis [23-25]. Of interest, we have recently observed that administration of the polyamine biosynthesis inhibitor alpha-difluoromethylornithine (DFMO) increased the secretion of IGF-binding proteins in some human breast cancer cell lines [14]. Thus, at least with regard to IGFs, polyamines could affect the action of these growth factors by influencing the secretion of their binding proteins.

Given the potentially important roles played by growth factors and polyamines in the control of breast cancer cell proliferation, it is conceivable that effective interference with these pathways may hold promise for the development of new treatment strategies in breast cancer. We will review here some experimental as well as preliminary clinical data providing support for this therapeutic approach.

Growth Factors as Targets for Antitumour Therapy

Somatostatin Analogue Therapy

The introduction of long-acting somatostatin analogues has been a major advance in the treatment of several functioning endocrine tumours [26,27]. Among these compounds octreotide has received the most extensive clinical testing and is currently FDA approved for treatment of Vipomas and the carcinoid syndrome. There are several potential mechanisms of antitumour action of somatostatin analogues in breast cancer. Suppression of circulating levels of IGF-I and EGF has been demonstrated in patients chronically treated with these drugs [28,29]. Furthermore, in different experimental systems, somatostatin has been shown to inhibit EGF action [30,31]. Somatostatin analogues could also exert a direct inhibitory effect on tumour growth as recently suggested *in vitro* in the MCF-7 breast cancer cell line [23]. The presence of somatostatin receptors in a significant fraction of human breast cancer specimens [33] provides support for this potential mechanism of antitumour action. Finally, these compounds could induce tumour regression by inhibition of growth hormone and under certain conditions prolactin release [34-38]. Consistent prolactin suppression can best be achieved by concomitant administration of dopaminergic drugs such as bromocriptine [28]. Although human breast cancer is predominantly oestrogen dependent, there is evidence in the literature that growth hormone and prolactin, both lactogenic in women, could stimulate breast cancer growth [39-41]. Octreotide, either alone or in combination with bromocriptine, has been tested in few pilot clinical trials, usually conducted in heavily pretreated women with advanced breast cancer [28,42-44]. Overall, these studies indicate that moderate suppression of growth hormone and somatomedin-C production can be achieved in most but not all patients. Thus, additional efforts need to be placed in determining the optimal schedule of administration of the drug to maximise its endocrine effects. Due to the heavy pretreatment in most patients, the therapeutic potential of somatostatin analogue therapy in advanced breast

Table 1. Summary of pilot clinical trials testing the role of octreotide in the treatment of advanced breast cancer

Author (ref.)	No. pts.	Treatment schedule	No. of responders	Duration of response	Endocrine effects
Manni et al. [28]	10	100-200 μg s.c. BID + bromocriptine 2.5 mg BID p.o.	1[a]	7 mos	- GH ↓ in 7/9 - Sm-C ↓ in 6/9 (~ 30%) - PRL ↓ in 8/9 - No effect on gonadotropins, oestrogens, cortisol, thyroid hormones
Vennin et al. [42]	14	100 μg s.c. BID	3[a]	4 mos [b]	-Sm-C ↓ in 8/12 (~ 30%)
Pollak et al. [43]	8[c]	400 μg s.c. TID	?	-	- ↓ GH - ↓ Sm-C (~ 50%)
Stolfi [44]	10	750 μg i.v. TID x 10 days -> 500 μg i.m. BID x 5 days	3[d]	e	- Endocrine studies not performed

a only disease stabilisation was observed in these patients
b treatment was discontinued in the absence of tumour regression despite lack of progression
c this group includes patients with pancreatic, ovarian, breast, kidney and colon cancer. The exact distribution of patients among the various tumour types was not reported
d all these patients were previously untreated
e duration of response not reported since the treatment was discontinued after 15 days

cancer cannot be adequately assessed. The only patients shown to have obtained objective tumour regression were previously untreated (Table 1). Following our published report, we have treated 7 additional patients with the combination of octreotide and bromocriptine. Of these, one obtained objective tumour regression consisting of a decrease in the size of metastatic skin lesions and healing of lytic bone metastasis for a 6-month duration.

Somatostatin analogue therapy with octreotide has generally been reported to be free of major side effects [26,27]. The majority of complaints are gastrointestinal and consist of abdominal pain, cramping, loose stools and steatorrhoea. These symptoms, however, are usually transient and frequently subside despite continuation of treatment. Glucose intolerance, when present, is mild and clinically insignificant [45-48]. Perhaps of more concern is the development of cholelithiasis, which has been reported in 4 of 9 patients with normal gallbladder before initiation of therapy after 12 months of octreotide treatment [49].

In view of the limited toxicity and encouraging endocrine effects, larger clinical trials should be conducted in less heavily pretreated patients to establish the therapeutic efficacy of somatostatin analogues either alone or in combination with standard therapy in the treatment of metastatic breast cancer.

Anti-Growth Factor Antibody Therapy

The development of neutralising antibodies directed against growth factors and/or their receptors offers potential for improved antitumour therapy in breast cancer. Numerous *in vitro* studies have demonstrated that, at least in the presence of serum, neutralisation of IGFs and TGF-alpha action with antibodies directed to the peptides or their receptors inhibits breast cancer growth in a variety of experimental systems [50-53]. More controversy exists regarding the antiproliferative effect of these antibodies in the absence of serum, thus raising some doubts on the role of endogenously produced growth factors, particularly as mediators of hormone action.

Whether inhibiting serum factors or endogenously produced peptides, anti-growth factor antibody therapy has been consistently shown to be effective in inhibiting breast cancer growth *in vitro* [50-53].
It is encouraging to observe that such treatment strategy is also effective *in vivo* in nude mice carrying human tumour xenografts. Masui et al. [54] have demonstrated that intraperitoneal administration of 2 anti-EGF receptor antibodies inhibited the growth of human A-431 tumours in athymic mice. A similar inhibition of tumour growth was observed with 3 additional cell lines which were also sensitive in culture but was not observed against other tumour cell lines that were not inhibited *in vitro*. Arteaga et al. [55] observed that administration of alpha-IR3, an anti-IGF-I receptor antibody, inhibited in a dose-dependent fashion the growth of the oestrogen-independent MDA-231 breast cancer cells in nude mice. In contrast, the growth of the oestrogen-dependent MCF-7 cells was unaffected, even though this cell line was growth-inhibited *in vitro*.
Of most interest, in a recent phase I clinical trial, Mendelsohn [56] has shown that a labelled anti-EGF receptor antibody was able to localise sites of squamous carcinoma of the lung which bear increased numbers of EGF-receptors. The data also indicated that patients tolerated the presence of saturating concentrations of the antibody in their blood for more than 3 days without significant toxicity. Taken together, these preliminary observations suggest that therapy with anti-receptor monoclonal antibodies is a worthwhile area for clinical investigation in the future.

Polyamines as Possible Targets for Antitumour Therapy

Following the observation that polyamines are essential mediators of hormonal effect on breast cancer cell proliferation *in vitro* [57-59], we have recently focused on their potential role as targets for antitumour therapy *in vivo*. We observed that administration of DFMO was able to completely abolish hormonal stimulation of tumour growth in ovariectomised NMU tumour bearing rats [60]. The specificity of the DFMO effect through the polyamine pathway was supported by the ability of exogenous putrescine administration to reverse at least in part the antiproliferative action of DFMO. DFMO administration, on the other hand, did not influence oestradiol stimulated progesterone receptor synthesis in the same tumours and uterine growth in the same animals [60]. Taken collectively, these results emphasise the selectivity of polyamine involvement in hormonal action despite demonstration of hormonal control of polyamine synthesis in virtually every endocrine target tissue tested so far. Such selectivity, if confined indeed to hormonal modulation of neoplastic cell growth, could represent a major therapeutic advantage in the use of anti-polyamine therapy in the treatment of human breast cancer.
In recent experiments, we have addressed the potential merit of combined hormone depletion and anti-polyamine therapy. In experiments again conducted in the NMU mammary tumour, we have observed that combined ovariectomy and DFMO induced a faster and greater suppression of the labelling indices of all cell types (glandular, myoepithelial, and non-epithelial cells) than the individual treatments [61]. Combination treatment also produced more profound morphologic changes consisting of a reduction in the fraction of glandular cells as well as a decrease in cell volume. The ability of combined manipulation of the hormone and polyamine pathway to rapidly influence tumour cell kinetics before even inducing any major change in tumour volume, may represent a significant step towards the implementation of kinetically targeted cytotoxic chemotherapy.
Recently, Carbone et al. [62] have conducted a phase I pharmacokinetic study of DFMO in patients with prostate, colorectal and bladder cancer. The authors observed that DFMO can be given orally for up to 6 months at a dose of 0.5 mg/m^2 daily without any significant toxicity. A >50% reduction in TPA-induced ornithine decarboxylase in skin punch biopsies was also documented to support the activity of the drug. These preliminary results offer hope for the potential future use of DFMO as an antitumour and possibly chemopreventive agent in humans.

Table 2. Novel approaches to the endocrine therapy of breast cancer

Agent	Comment
New antioestrogens	Less oestrogen agonistic effect
New aromatase inhibitors	More selectivity for the aromatase enzyme (and fewer side effects)
GnRH antagonists	Elimination of the flare phenomenon
High-dose progestins	Superior antitumour action compared to conventional doses. Beneficial effect on cachexia
Antiprogestins	? Induction of terminal differentiation and cell death. Adrenal insufficiency is a significant side effect
Vitamin D analogues	Differentiating agents with less hypercalcaemic effect

Conclusions

We have discussed here potential future approaches to the treatment of breast cancer on the basis of emerging new information on the basic mechanisms controlling breast cancer cell proliferation. Additional lines of investigation not covered here are currently being pursued in the attempt to improve the endocrine treatment of this malignancy [63]. They are outlined in Table 2. In my opinion, it is unlikely that any of the treatments discussed or listed in Table 2 will significantly prolong survival in patients with metastatic breast cancer. Demonstration, however, of efficacy in this setting would create a rationale for testing these therapies in women with early disease with the hope of increasing the still small benefit on overall survival currently provided by adjuvant therapy.

Acknowledgement

This work is supported by a grant from the National Cancer Institute, PO1 CA40011.

REFERENCES

1 Santen RJ, Manni A, Harvey H and Redmond C: Endocrine treatment of breast cancer in women. Endo Rev 1990 (11):221-265
2 Henderson IC, Canellos GP: Cancer of the breast. N Engl J Med 1980 (302):17-30
3 Osborne CK, Coronado EB, Kitten LH, Arteaga CI, Fuqua SAW, Ramasharma K, Marshall M and Li CH: Insulin-like growth factor-II (IGF-II): a potential autocrine/paracrine growth factor for human breast cancer acting via the IGF-I receptor. Molec Endocrinol 1989 (3):1701-1709
4 Huff KK, Knabbe C, Lindsey R, Kaufman D, Bronzert D, Lippman ME and Dickson RB: Multihormonal regulation of insulin-like growth factor-I-related protein in MCF-7 human breast cancer cells. Molec Endocrinol 1988 (2):200-208
5 Bates SE, Davidson NE, Valverius EM, Freter CE, Dickson RB, Tam JP, Kudlow JE, Lippman ME and Salomons DS: Expression of transforming growth factor alpha and its messenger ribonucleic acid in human breast cancer: its regulation by estrogen and its possible functional significance. Molec Endocrinol 1988 (2):543-555
6 Knabbe C, Lippman ME, Wakefield LM, Flanders KC, Kasid A, Derynck R and Dickson RB: Evidence that transforming growth factor-ß is a hormonally regulated negative growth factor in human breast cancer cells. Cell 1987 (48):417-428
7 Stewart AJ, Johnson MD, May FEB and Westley BR: Role of insulin-like growth factors and the type I insulin-like growth factor receptor in the estrogen-stimulated proliferation of human breast cancer cells. J Biol Chem 1990 (265):21172-21178
8 Osborne CK, Hamilton B and Nover M: Receptor binding and processing of epidermal growth factor by human breast cancer cells. J Clin Endocrinol Metab 1982 (55):86-93
9 Osborne CK, Hamilton B, Titus G and Livingston RB: Epidermal growth factor stimulation of human breast cancer cells in culture. Cancer Res 1980 (40):2361-2366
10 Yee D, Paik S, Lebovic R, Favoni R, Cullen K, Lippman ME and Rosen N: Analysis of IGF-I gene expression in malignancy - evidence for a paracrine role in human breat cancer. Molec Endocrinol 1989 (3):509-517
11 Bronzert DA, Pantazis P, Antoniades HN, Kasid A, Davidson N, Dickson RB and Lippman ME: Synthesis and secretion of platelet-derived growth factor by human breast cancer cell lines. Proc Natl Acad Sci USA 1987 (84):5763-5767
12 De Leon DD, Baker B, Wilson DM, Lamson G and Rosenfeld RG: Insulin-like growth factor binding proteins in human breast cancer cells: relationship to hIGFBP-2 and hIGFBP-3. J Clin Endocrinol Metab 1990 (71):530-532
13 De Leon DD, Wilson SM, Baker B, Lamson G, Hintz RL and Rosenfeld RG: Characterization of insulin-like growth factor binding proteins from human breast cancer cells. Molec Endocrinol 1989 (3):567-574
14 Kim I, Manni A, Lynch J and Hammond JM: Identification and regulation of insulin-like growth factor binding proteins produced by hormone-dependent and -independent human breast cancer cell lines. Molec Cell Endocrinol 1991 (780):71-78
15 Elgin RG, Busby WH Jr and Clemmons DR: An insulin-like growth factor (IGF) binding protein enhances the biologic response to IGF-I. Proc Natl Acad Sci USA 1987 (84):3254-3258
16 Blum WF, Jenne EW, Reppin F, Kietzmann K, Ranke BM and Bierich JR: Insulin-like growth factor I (IGF-I)-binding protein complex is a better mitogen than free IGF-I. Endocrinology 1989 (125):766-772
17 Thomas T, Kiang DT: Structural alterations and stabilization of rabbit uterine estrogen receptors by natural polyamines. Cancer Res 1987 (47):1799-1804
18 Thomas T, Kiang DT: Modulation of the binding of progesterone receptor to DNA by polyamines. Cancer Res 1988 (48):1217-1222
19 Manni A, Wright C, Feil P, Baranao L, Demers L, Garcia M and Rochefort H: Autocrine stimulation by estradiol-regulated growth factors of rat hormone-responsive mammary cancer: interaction with the polyamine pathway. Cancer Res 1986 (46):1594-1598
20 Manni A, Wright C, Hsu C-J and Hammond JM: Polyamines and autocrine control of tumor growth by prolactin in experimental breast cancer in culture. Endocrinology 1986 (119):2033-2037
21 Glikman PL, Manni A, Bartholomew M and Demers L: Polyamine involvement in basal and estradiol-stimulated insulin-like growth factor I secretion and action in breast cancer cell lines in culture. J Steroid Biochem Molec Biol 1990 (37):1-10
22 Kim I, Manni A, Lynch J and Demers L: Polyamine involvement in the secretion and action of TGF-alpha in hormone sensitive human breast cancer cells in culture. Breast Cancer Res Treat 1991 (18):83-91
23 Manni A, Wright C, Luk GD, Davis G and Demers L: Role of polyamines in the synthesis of estradiol-regulated growth factors in rat mammary cancer in culture. Breast Cancer Res Treat 1987 (9):45-51
24 Manni A, Badger B, Wright C, Ahman SR, Santner SJ and Luk G: Role of polyamines in the synthesis of prolactin-regulated growth factors by experimental breast cancer in culture. Breast Cancer Res Treat 1987 (10):191-196
25 Cohen FJ, Manni A, Glikman P, Bartholomew M and Demers L: Interactions between growth factor secretion and polyamines in MCF-7 breast cancer cells. Eur J Cancer 1990 (26):255-273
26 Katz MD and Erstad BL: Octreotide, a new somatostatin analogue. Clin Pharm 1989 (8):255-273
27 Gorden P, Comi RJ, Maton PN and Go VLW: Somatostatin and somatostatin analogue (SMS 201-995) in treatment of hormone-secreting tumors of the pituitary and gastrointestinal tract and non-neoplastic diseases of the gut. Ann Int Med 1989 (110):35-50
28 Manni A, Boucher AE, Demers LM, Harvey HA, Lipton A, Simmonds MA and Bartholomew M: Endocrine effects of combined somatostatin analog and bromocriptine therapy in women with advanced

breast cancer. Breast Cancer Res Treat 1989 (14):289-298
29 Chirlanda G, Ucciolo L, Perri F, Altomonte L, Bertoi A, Manna R, Frati L and Greco AU: Epidermal growth factor, somatostatin and psoriasis. Lancet 1983 (i):65
30 Viguerie N, Tahiri-Jouti N, Ayral AM, Cambillau C, Scemama JL, Bastie MJ, Knuhtsen S, Esteve JP, Pradayrol L, Susini C and Vaysse N: Direct inhibitory effects of a somatostatin analog, SMS 201-995, on AR4-2J cell proliferation via pertussis toxin-sensitive guanosine triphosphate-binding protein independent mechanism. Endocrinology 1989 (124):1017-1025
31 Mascardo RN and Sherline P: Somatostatin inhibits rapid intrasomal separation and cell proliferation induced by epidermal growth factor. Endocrinology 1982 (111):1394-1396
32 Setyono-Han B, Henkelman MS, Foekens JA and Klihn JGM: Direct inhibitory effects of somatostatin (analogues) on thre growth of human breast cancer cells. Cancer Res 1987 (47):1566-1570
33 Reubi JC, Waser B, Foekens JA, Klihn JGM, Lamberts SWJ and Laissue J: Somatostatin receptor incidence and distribution in breast cancer using receptor autoradiography: relationship to EGF receptors. Int J Cancer 1990 (46):416-420
34 Schally AV, Coy DH and Meyers CA: Hypothalamic regulatory hormones. Ann Rev Biochem 1978 (47):89-128
35 Schally AV and Redding TW: Somatostatin analogs as adjuncts to agonists of luteinizing hormone-releasing hormone in the treatment of experimental prostate cancer. Proc Natl Acad Sci USA 1987 (84):7275-7279
36 Schally AV, Cai RZ, Torres-Aleman I, Redding TW, Szoke B, Fu D, Hierowski MT, Colaluca J and Konturek S: Endocrine, gastrointestinal and antitumor activity of somatostatin analogs. In: Moody TW (ed) Neural and Endocrine Peptides and Receptors. Plenum Publ Corp, New York 1986 pp 73-83
37 Schally AV, Redding TW, Cai RZ, Paz JI, Ben-David M and Comaru-Schally AM: Somatostatin analogs in the treatment of various experimental tumors. In: Klijn JGM (ed) International Symposium on Hormonal Manipulation of Cancer: Peptides, Growth Factors and New (anti)Steroidal Agents. Raven Press, New York 1987 pp 431-440
38 Schally AV, Redding TW, Paz-Bouza JI, Comaru-Schally AM and Mathe G: Current concept for improving treatment of prostate cancer based on combination of LH-RH agonists with other agents. In: Murphy GP, Khoury S, Kuss R, Chatelain C, Denis L (eds) Prostate Cancer, Part A. Alan R Liss, New York 1987 pp 173-197
39 Manni A, Wright C, Davis G, Glenn J, Joehl R and Feil P: Promotion by prolactin of the growth of human breast neoplasms cultured in vitro on the soft agar clonogenic assay. Cancer Res 1986 (46):1669-1672
40 Malarkey WB, Kennedy M, Allred LE and Milo G: Physiological concentrations of prolactin can promote the growth of human breast tumor cells in culture. J Clin Endocrinol Metab 1983 (56):673-677
41 DeSouza I, Morgan L, Lewis UJ, Raggatt PR, Salih H and Hobbs JR: Growth-hormone dependence among human breast cancers. The Lancet 1974 (2):182-184
42 Vennin PH, Peyrat JP, Bonneterre J, Louchez MM, Harris AG and Demaile A: Effect of the long-acting somatostatin analogue SMS 201-995 (Sandostatin) in advanced breast cancer. Anticancer Res 1989 (9):153-156
43 Pollak MN, Polychronakos C and Guyda H: Somatostatin analogue SMS 201-995 reduces serum IGF-I levels in patients with neoplasms potentially dependent on IGF-I. Anticancer Res 1989 (9):889-892
44 Stolfi R, Parisi AM, Natoli C and Iacobelli S: Advanced breast cancer: response to somatostatin. Anticancer Res 1990 (10):203-204
45 Kvols KL, Moertel CG, O'Connell MJ, Schutt AJ, Rubin J and Hahn RJ: Treatment of the malignant carcinoid syndrome. Evaluation of a long-acting somatostatin analogue. N Engl J Med 1986 (315):663-666
46 Kvols LK, Buck M, Moertel CG, Schutt AJ, Rubin J, O'Connell MJ and Hahn RG: Treatment of metastatic islet cell carcinoma with a somatostatin analogue (SMS 201-995). Ann Int Med 1987 (107):162-168
47 Boden G, Ryan IG, Eisenschmid BL, Shelmet JJ and Owen OE: Treatment of inoperable glucagonoma with the long-acting somatostatin analogue SMS 201-995. N Engl J Med 1986 (314):1686-1689
48 Maton PN, O'Dorisio TM, Howe BA, McArthur KE, Howard JH, Cherner JA, Malarkey TB, Collen MJ, Gardner JD and Jensen RT: Effect of a long-acting somatostatin analogue (SMS 201-995) in a patient with pancreatic cholera. N Engl J Med 1985 (312):17-21
49 Ho KY, Weissberger AJ, Marbach P and Lazarus L: Therapeutic efficacy of the somatostatin analog SMS 201-995 (octroitide) in acromegaly: effects of dose and frequency and long-term safety. Ann Int Med 1990 (112):173-181
50 Arteaga CL and Osborne CK: Growth inhibition of human breast cancer cells in vitro with an antibody against the type I somatomedin receptor. Cancer Res 1989 (49):6237-6241
51 Ennis BW, Valverius EM, Bates SE, Lippman ME, Bellot F, Kris R, Schlessinger J, Masui H, Goldenberg A, Menselsohn J and Dickson RB: Anti-epidermal growth factor receptor antibodies inhibit the autocrine-stimulated growth of MDA-468 human breast cancer cells. Molec Endocrinol 1989 (3):1830-1838
52 Ahmed SR, Badger B, Wright C and Manni A: Role of transforming growth factor alpha in basal and hormone stimulated growth by estradiol, prolactin and progesterone in human and rat mammary tumor cells: studies using TGF-alpha and EGF receptor antibodies. J Steroid Biochem Molec Biol 1991 (38):687-693
53 Glickman PL, Manni A, Bartholomew M and Demers L: Polyamine involvement in basal and estradiol-stimulated insulin-like growth factor I secretion and action in breast cancer cells in culture. J Steroid Biochem Molec Biol 1990 (37):1-10

54 Masui H, Kawamoto T, Sato JD, Wolf B, Sato GH and Mendelsohn J: Growth inhibition of human tumor cells in athymic mice by anti-EGF receptor monoclonal antibodies. Cancer Res 1984 (44):1002-1007
55 Arteaga CL, Kitten LJ, Coronado EB, Jacobs S, Full FC, Allred DC and Osborne CK: Blockade of the type I somatomedin receptor inhibits growth of human breast cancer cells in athymic mice. J Clin Invest 1989 (84):1418-1423
56 Mendelsohn J: Anti-epidermal growth factor receptor monoclonal antibodies as potential anti-cancer agents. J Steroid Biochem Molec Biol 1990 (37):889-892
57 Manni A and Wright C: Polyamines as mediators of estrogen action on the growth of experimental breast cancer in rats. JNCI 1984 (73):511-514
58 Manni A and Wright C: Polyamines as mediators of the effect of prolactin and growth hormone on the growth of N-nitroso-N-methylurea-induced rat mammary tumor culture in vitro in soft agar. JNCI 1985 (74):941-944
59 Lima G and Shiu RPC: Role of polyamines in estradiol-induced growth of human breast cancer cells. Cancer Res 1985 (45):2466-2470
60 Manni A, Badger B, Lynch J and Demers L: Selectivity of polyamine involvement in hormone action on normal and neoplastic target tissues of the rat. Breast Cancer Res Treat 1990 (17):187-196
61 Manni A, Lancaster S, English H, Badger B, Lynch J and Demers L: Kinetic and morhopmetric response of heterogeneous populations of NMU-induced rat mammary tumor cells to hormone and antipolyamine therapy in vivo. Breast Cancer Res Treat 1990 (17):179-186
62 Carbone PP, Love RR, Carey P, Tutsch K, Verma AK, Wilding G and Silmore-Cunningham D: Phase I and pharmacokinetics study of difluoromethyl-ornithine (DFMO), a potential chemopreventive. Proc of the 82nd Mtg of the Am Assoc Cancer Res, May 15-18, 1991, Houston, Texas. (abstr 1209)
63 Dowsett M: Novel approaches to the endocrine therapy of breast cancer. Eur J Cancer 1990 (26):989-992

Prognostic Factors in Primary Breast Cancer: Second Thoughts

Susan M. Thorpe [1] and Carsten Rose [2]

1 Department of Tumour Endocrinology, The Fibiger Institute, Ndr. Frihavnsgade 70, 2100 Copenhagen, Denmark (sponsored by the Danish Cancer Society)
2 Department of Oncology R, Odense University Hospital, Sdr. Boulevard 29, 5000 Odense, Denmark

Adjuvant treatment of primary breast cancer is now generally accepted to be of significant value in specific subgroups of patients at high risk for recurrent disease. As the incidence of breast cancer continues to rise, the interest in finding new characteristics associated with good versus poor prognosis is increasing. While the literature abounds with reports of potentially interesting tumour markers, in most clinical settings the traditional pathological features described at the time of primary surgery remain the main criteria for distinguishing between patients who should versus those who should not receive adjuvant therapy. Steroid hormone receptor profiles are an exception to this rule. Receptor status has recently been incorporated into the matrix of variables used to make the above distinction in a number of centres. Yet even for the oestrogen receptor, the eldest of the biochemical tumour markers currently gaining recognition as a prognostic factor, one still finds dissent in the literature as to whether steroid hormone receptor determinations are useful and how they should be implemented in the clinical management of primary breast cancer.
Since reviews summarising the multitude of potentially interesting prognostic factors are already available in the literature [1], we will not present such a review here. Instead, we will give possible reasons that may help in understanding why it appears to be so difficult to identify and verify novel prognostic factors. In so doing, we will draw upon historical examples of investigations specifically regarding steroid hormone receptor determinations and their potential clinical relevance to illustrate our points.

Politics of Clinically Relevant Research

Research funding situations in society demand result-oriented projects. The number and timing of publications are commonly accepted measures of productivity and originality. Generally, it is more prestigious to be among the first to publish new concepts within a given field, and, due to weaknesses in the system itself, quantity rather than quality often carries more weight. These forces interact to encourage the reseacher to publish results as early as possible. This effect can be detrimental to furthering "knowledge": results drawn from investigations conducted on populations that are heterogeneous, too small, or have too few "events" are frequently unreproducible. Such results tend to confuse rather than clarify the overall view. It is against this background that the complexity of establishing the usefulness of novel prognostic factors becomes understandable.

Definition of the Term "Prognostic Factor"

While the definition of "prognostic factor" can be the subject of interesting semantic discussion, there are basically two different clinical situations in which it is commonly used. The first is that in which the natural course of the disease is considered, while the second is that in which a potential benefit of adjuvant therapy is evaluated. In this chapter we reserve the term "prognosis" for the former situation and employ the term "prediction" for the latter. Surprisingly few studies are found in the literature that distinguish between prognosis and prediction. Often a mishmash of patients - some of whom are treated and some who are not treated with adjuvant therapy - is presented in the same analysis.

Experimental Approaches to Discovering and Defining Novel Prognostic Factors

Having determined that a particular factor might be of potential prognostic and/or predictive value, the next step commonly taken in elucidating its possible use is to compare the occurrence and/or expression of the factor among patients with a high risk for recurrent disease with those at low risk. If a difference is found, the next step often entails a larger-scale, retrospective investigation of a group of primary breast cancer patients. Results from such investigations are usually presented first in a univariate form, while more thorough investigations examine the factor of interest in a multivariate analysis encompassing established prognostic factors. It is this more comprehensive multivariate analysis which is able to address the question of whether the proposed prognostic factor is indeed of independent significance or merely reflects aspects of pre-existing, established prognostic factors. Provided that the proposed novel factor *is* observed to be of significant value, and pending confirmation of these results in other independent collaborative studies, it then becomes reasonable to incorporate the new prognostic factor in a prospective study.

Carefully designed protocols may curtail what otherwise would be a considerable lag phase between the time of the primary investigation and a subsequent study testing the validity of the original results. For example, if a large enough patient population is studied, the population can be randomly divided into two equal groups prior to the primary data analysis. The results and conclusions generated from the analysis of the primary set can then be rapidly tested on the supplemental set of patients.

Most prospective studies are necessarily multi-institutional. Several methodological prerequisites should be met before prospective studies utilising a new prognostic/predictive factor are initiated. Primary among these is standardisation of the assay method for determining the factor. Equally important, the assay method must be under continual intra- and inter-laboratory quality control to screen for potential errors. Such quality-control programmes ensure that the assay results generated from the different institutions can be pooled and used for a meaningful analysis of the data.

Given the simple, direct nature of the approach outlined above, why then does it remain so difficult to discover and validate new prognostic factors? Part of the explanation lies in the nature of breast cancer itself. Although the risk of developing breast cancer increases with age, it is a disease that is observed even in women under 30 years of age. Moreover, breast cancer is a disease recognised to be associated with an individual's reproductive history. It is, therefore, not surprising that breast cancer is a multi-faceted disease and might lend itself more easily to investigation when grouped into natural subdivisions (e.g., menopausal status of the patient). In view of this fact, clinical adjuvant treatment protocols often differ for pre- and postmenopausal patients. Nevertheless, in the zealous search for novel prognostic factors, biologically relevant subgrouping of patients is too often ignored.

In academical terms, the reasonableness of studying specific, well-defined patient groups with regard to treatment regimens and menopausal status can probably be agreed upon. Practically, these criteria can be met only in large collaborative studies which, unfortunately, are few in number.

The experience of the Danish Breast Cancer Cooperative Group (DBCG) effectively illustrates the above-mentioned points. The DBCG constitutes a collaborative, nationwide project initiated in 1977 that registers 95% of the primary breast cancer cases in Denmark; its goal is to enter as many patients as possible in the adjuvant treatment programme in order to improve survival of breast cancer, and simultaneously enhance the knowledge of the disease [2]. Steroid hormone receptor determinations were already professed to be of potential predictive value at the inception of the DBCG programme and were, therefore, included as widely as possible in the trials. Initially, for logistic reasons, only hospitals within a geographically defined area were encouraged to forward tissue to a central laboratory for receptor analysis. As the study progressed and the interest in the project peaked, a larger number of institutions began sending tissue for analysis. At present, tissue is sent for biochemical receptor analysis from approximately 90% of the departments participating in the DBCG programme. Biochemical receptor determinations were performed on 15% of the patients in the early years of the trials and are now provided for approximately 40% of the patients.

In the period between 24 August, 1979 and 31 December, 1989, a total of 7,259 primary breast cancer biopsies were forwarded from departments within the geographically defined area to a single receptor laboratory. Only 4,332 of the patients (60%) fulfilled the criteria stipulated in the entrance requirements for participation in the adjuvant treatment protocols (Table 1).

The importance of collecting sufficient numbers of patients to address specific questions has been noted above. As can be seen in Table 1, an initially very large number of patients rapidly diminishes when women are grouped according to menopausal status and treatment regime. For example, referring to Table 1, if the goal is to evaluate the possible role of receptor determinations for prognosis (i.e., no adjuvant treatment) among the premenopausal patients, only 13% of the total population of protocolled primary breast cancer patients is available for study. This corresponds to only 8% of all primary breast cancer biopsies analysed for receptor content.

Not only are adequate numbers of patients required before one can reasonably attempt to address questions regarding the potential value of various factors in predicting disease outcome, but the median time of observation is also a critical element since the statistical validity of clinical analyses is based upon the number of events observed. Again, the nature of the disease itself works against rather than for us: breast cancer can lie dormant for years before manifesting itself again. Especially in studies on the low-risk group where the 5-year rate of recurrence/death is typically 25-35%, a median observation time of at least 5 years is desirable to minimise the skewing effects of late recurrence.

Few published studies fulfill these fairly simple criteria for valid investigation of potential prognostic factors. Taken together with the comments regarding the political nature of clinical research noted above, it is not surprising that reports in the literature constitute a multitude of studies of small populations of heterogeneous patient groups, most of which have sub-optimal observation periods. It is then no wonder that such conclusions as can be gathered from the literature tend to confuse rather than clarify the questions at hand.

Table 1. Distribution of 4,332 patients protocolled in the DBCG project with steroid hormone receptor determinations: Experience of a single receptor laboratory

			Menopausal status		
Protocol[1]	Risk group	Adjuvant treatment	pre-	peri-	post-
a	low	none	548	243	1218
b	high	yes	780	317	0
c	high	yes	0	0	1226

1 Patients protocolled in both 77- and 82- generations of DBCG protocols are included

Are Steroid Receptors of Significant Prognostic and/or Predictive Value?

Let us now, against this background, recapitulate the experiences surrounding the question of whether oestrogen and progesterone receptor analyses constitute independent prognostic and/or predictive factors in primary breast cancer.

One of the earliest reports ascribing a possible prognostic value to oestrogen receptors was presented in 1977 and was based on an investigation of 145 primary breast cancer patients of all ages, approximately 68% of whom were treated with adjuvant treatment modalities [3]. The median time of observation was 18 months. On the basis of our present knowledge, it is reasonable to assume that the significant difference observed in disease-free survival between oestrogen receptor (ER)-positive versus ER-negative patients is largely due to an association between presence of ER and benefit of endocrine therapy modalities. It has taken us almost 15 more years of research to arrive at what appears to be a consensus regarding the association between ER status and potential benefit of adjuvant endocrine therapy [4]! Equally shocking is the fact that there is as yet no consensus on the question whether receptor analyses can be used to define a subgroup of patients who are deemed to be at such low risk of recurrent disease that they can be spared adjuvant therapeutic intervention subsequent to surgery. This lack of consensus is not due to a shortage of publications on the subject. Consultation of the Medline literature search database reveals that no fewer than 304 publications with a combination of the 3 key words, "breast neoplasms/prognosis/oestrogen receptors" have appeared between 1987 and mid 1991.

Having access to one of the largest known unselected data bases of primary breast cancer patients, what have we learned from the DBCG trials? At a median observation time of approximately 35 months, it was possible in 1984 to observe that the potential benefit of adjuvant tamoxifen therapy among 291 postmenopausal patients was greatest among those ER-positive patients with the highest levels of ER [5]. These early observations have since been confirmed in an even larger group of postmenopausal DBCG patients [6] and are in accordance with the results seen in the EBCTCG study [4].

Analysis of the potential role that ER and/or progesterone receptor (PgR) might play in the natural history of the disease required a longer observation time. At a median follow-up of 50 months, we analysed the potential role of ER and PgR in patients not treated with adjuvant modalities [7]. Among the 807 low-risk patients available for the study, a complex situation was observed. If all 807 patients were considered simultaneously, as often has been the case in the literature, a significant but small (~8% at 3 yrs) difference in recurrence-free survival (RFS) was observed with regard to PgR but not ER (Table 2). However, when the patients were subdivided according to menopausal status, much greater differences in RFS between receptor-positive and receptor-negative groups were observed for both ER and PgR (~14% and ~24%, respectively, at 3 yrs) in pre- but not postmenopausal patients. In the postmenopausal group, the RFS curves for receptor-positive and receptor-negative patients were almost superimposed.

At the time we conducted our investigation, there were only 2 other investigations found in the literature that included at least 500 patients, none of whom received adjuvant therapy [8,9] (Table 2). A significantly longer RFS was found for ER-positive patients in one study [8], while no difference was found in the other [9]. The former study most closely resembles our own in that the frequency of ER positivity was found to be 74% (frequency of ER+ in our own study = 75%), while the comparable figure from the latter study is 46%. The discrepancy in the findings of these 3 studies points to one of the essential caveats when analysing the potential usefulness of steroid hormone receptor determinations: steroid hormone receptor determinations are notoriously difficult to standardise [10].

The frequencies of receptor positivity reported in the literature vary from 46% [21] to 76% [22] for ER and from 45% [23] to 68% [24] for PgR. In general, studies revealing differences between RFS for receptor-positive and receptor-negative patients tend to have the higher frequencies of receptor positivity (Table 2). Moreover, within the DBCG project we have demonstrated that inclusion of data from sub-

Table 2. Studies of RFS according to ER status among node-negative breast cancer patients who have not received systemic adjuvant therapy

First author [ref]	No.	% ER+	Follow-up	Comments regarding RFS
Cooke [11]	166	55	mean, 19 mo	advantage ER+; $p < 0.01$
Crowe [8]	510	74	median, 51 mo	advantage ER+; $p < 0.03$
Sears [12]	155	76	max, 72 mo	advantage ER+; NS[1]
Mason [13]	224	58	median, 38 mo	advantage ER+; NS
Alanko [14]	131	55	mean, 41 mo	advantage ER+; NS
Valagussa [15]	464	71	median, 60 mo	advantantage ER+; $p < 0.0001$
Butler [9]	556	46	median, 75 mo	NS
Adami [16]	94	70	89% pts, >36 mo	advantage ER+; $p < 0.05$
Howat [17]	99	58	min, 58 mo	NS
Caldarola [18]	126	38	median, 49 mo	NS
Thorpe [7]	803	75	median, 50 mo	advantage ER+; NS overall; < 0.001 for premenopausal
Fisher [19]	825	64	5 yr	advantage ER+; $p < 0.005$
Courdi [20]	167	60	analysed at 8 yrs	advantage ER+; $p < 0.03$

1 NS: not significant

optimally performed receptor analyses together with data from optimally performed receptor analyses substantially reduces the ability to distinguish between RFS of receptor-positive and receptor-negative patients [25].

Apart from its importance to the validity of the results, the problem of the duration of the observation time manifests itself in yet another manner when analysing the data. While whatever factor is being measured (e.g., receptor concentration) may be an intrinsic trait of the tumour, the effect of which may persist in influencing the course of the disease, it is equally conceivable that what is being measured may represent a transient characteristic, the effect of which may be lost in time. Thus, the initial ability of receptor status to distinguish between good and poor prognostic and/or predictive groups may disappear with time.

With the large number of patients and the prolonged observation time now attained, the potential role of ER in the natural history of postmenopausal, primary breast cancer is finally becoming apparent. We found it puzzling that neither ER nor PgR status appeared to be significantly associated with the natural history of the disease in the older patients in the DBCG study. For further clarification, we re-analysed this particular patient group in a less traditional manner: patients were subdivided into 3 rather than 2 categories according to ER concentration. To our amazement we found that postmenopausal patients with the highest ER concentrations had a RFS as poor as that of the ER-negative patients [6]. This observation is based on a population of 952 patients with a recurrence/mortality rate of 24% and should, therefore, be reasonably certain. Nevertheless, we eagerly await results from similar investigations to see whether the finding will be confirmed.

In summary, despite nearly 20 years of re-

search on ER in relation to clinical outcome, we have only in the most recent years become able to define reliably the association between receptor content in the primary tumour and both the natural history and the early course of adjuvantly treated disease.
Klijn and Foekens' recent review [1] concerning prognostic factors and breast cancer gives a comprehensive summary of the multitude of other potentially valuable prognostic and predictive factors that are currently being considered. These factors cover a broad spectrum of characteristics reflective of various aspects of tumour biology. They include markers of differentiation (surface antigens, e.g., CA 15.3), growth factor receptors (EGFR), measures of cell proliferation kinetics (DNA ploidy, S-phase, Ki-67, thymidine labelling index), signs of metastatic potential (concentrations of proteolytic enzymes, e.g., cathepsin D, uPA), genetic changes (chromosomal deletions/rearrangements), and indications of transformation (oncogenes). The results of studies published on most of these factors are important for generating hypotheses and designing new investigations. Due to relatively small patient numbers and/or short observation times in the existing studies, the results - with few exceptions - cannot yet be considered conclusive.

Future Perspectives

Ideally, we should aim at establishing a "prognostic index", an algorithm that incorporates the known risk hazards associated with recognised prognostic/predictive factors. By applying this algorithm to the individual patient, the clinician would have a means by which to evaluate whatever therapeutic modality is best suited for the patient. Apart from the psychological and medical importance such an approach would have for the individual patient, its potential societal and economic impact on the management of cancer is clear. Although it may seem utopian, a similar approach is currently employed with reasonable success in at least one centre [26,27].
Responsible, serious research is needed on a widespread basis to attain the above goal. Prudent use of material deposited in "tumour banks" according to well-designed experimental protocols can facilitate more rapid advancement than has been experienced in clarifying the potential usefulness of steroid hormone receptors for the treatment of breast cancer.

REFERENCES

1 Klijn JGM, Foekens JA: Prognostic factors in breast cancer. In: Goldhirsch A (ed) Endocrine Therapy of Breast Cancer IV. European School of Oncology Monograph Series. Springer-Verlag, Heidelberg 1990 pp 17-30

2 Andersen KW, Mouridsen HT, Castberg TH et al: Organization of the Danish adjuvant trials in breast cancer. Dan Med Bull 1981 (28):102-106

3 Knight WA, Livingstone RB, Gregory ER, McGurie WL: Estrogen receptor as an independent prognostic factor for early recurrence in breast cancer. Cancer Res 1977 (37):4667-4671

4 Early Breast Cancer Trialists' Collaborative Group (EBCTCG): Treatment of Early Breast Cancer. Oxford University Press, Oxford, 1990

5 Rose C, Thorpe SM, Andersen KW, Pedersen BV, Mouridsen HT, Blichert-Toft M, Rasmussen BB: Beneficial effect of adjuvant tamoxifen therapy in primary breast cancer patients wtih high estrogen receptor values. Lancet 1985 (i): 16-19

6 Thorpe SM, Christensen IJ, Rasmussen BB, Rose C: Short recurrence-free survival associated with high estrogen receptor levels in the natural history of postmenopausal, primary breast cancer. Submitted for publication

7 Thorpe SM, Rose C, Rasmussen BB, Mouridsen HT, Bayer T, Keiding N: Prognostic value of steroid hormone receptors: Multivariate analysis of systemically untreated patients with node negative primary breast cancer. Cancer Res 1987 (47): 6126-6133

8 Crowe JP, Hubay CA, Pearson OH, Marshall JS, Rosenblatt J, Mansour EG, Hermann RE, Jones JC, Flynne WJ, McGuire WL and participating investigators: Estrogen receptor status as a prognostic indicator for stage I breast cancer patients. Breast Cancer Res Treat 1982 (2):171-176

9 Butler JA, Bretsky S, Mendex-Botet C, Kinne DW: Estrogen receptor protein of breast cancer as a predictor or recurrence. Cancer 1985 (55):1178-1181

10 Thorpe SM: Steroid receptors in breast cancer: Sources of inter-laboratory variation in dextran-coated charcoal assays. Breast Cancer Res Treat 1987 (9):175-189

11 Cooke T, George D, Shields R, Maynard R, Griffiths K: Oestrogen receptors and prognosis in early breast cancer. Lancet 1979 (i):995-997

12 Sears HF, Janus C, Levy W, Hopson R, Crrech R, Grotzinger P: Breast cancer without axillary metastases. Are there high-risk biologic subpopulations? Cancer (Philadelphia) 1982 (50):1820-1827

13 Mason BH, Holdaway, KM, Mullins PR, Yee, LH, Kay RG: Progesterone and estrogen receptors as prognostic variables in breast cancer. Cancer Res 1983 (43):2985-2990

14 Alanko A, Heinonen E, Scheinin TM, Tolppanen EM, Vihko R: Oestrogen and progesterone receptors and disease-free interval in primary breast cancer. Br J Cancer 1984 (50):667-672

15 Valagussa P, Bignami P, Buzzoni R, DiFronzo G, Andreola S, Rilke F, Bonadonna G, Veronesi U: Are estrogen receptors alone a reliable prognostic factor in node negative breast cancer? In: Jones SE and Salmon SE (eds) Adjuvant Therapy of Cancer IV. Grune and Stratton Inc, London 1984 pp 407-515

16 Adami HO, Graffman S, Lindgren A, Sällström J: Prognostic implication of estrogen receptor content in breast cancer. Breast Cancer Res Treat 1985 (5):293-300

17 Howat JMT, Harris M, Swindell R, Barnes DM: The effect of estrogen and progesterone receptors on recurrence and survival in patients with carcinoma of the breast. Br J Cancer 1985 (51):263-270

18 Caldarola L, Volterrani P, Calderola B, Lai M, Jayme A, Gaglia P: The influence of hormone receptors and hormonal adjuvant therapy on disease-free survival in breast cancer: a multifactoral analysis. Eur J Cancer Clin Oncol 1986 (22):151-155

19 Fisher B, Redmond C, Fisher ER, Caplan R et al: Relative worth of estrogen or progesterone receptor and pathologic characteristics of differentiation as indicators of prognosis in node negative breast cancer patients: findings from National Surgical Adjuvant Breast and Bowel Project Protocol B-06. J Clin Oncol 1988 (6):1076-1087

20 Courdi A, Héry M, Dahan E, Gioanni J, Abbes M, Monticelli J, Ettore F, Moll J-L, Namer M: Factors affecting relapse in node-negative breast cancer. A multivariate analysis including labeling index. Eur J Cancer Clin Oncol 1989 (25):351-356

21 Poulsen HS: In-vitro tests and hormonal treatment of breast cancer. Prog Surg Path 1983 (5): 5-37

22 Pinchon MF, Pallud C, Brunet M, Milgrom E: Relationship of presence of progesterone receptors to prognosis in early breast cancer. Cancer Res 1980 (40): 3357-3360

23 Martin PM, Rolland PH, Jacquemier J, Rolland AM, Toga M: Multiple steroid receptors in human breast cancer. II. Estrogen and progestin receptors in 672 primary tumors. Cancer Chemother Pharmacol 1979 (2):107-113

24 Thorpe SM, Rose C, Pedersen BV, Rasmussen BB: Estrogen and progesterone receptor profile patterns in primary breast cancer. Breast Cancer Res Treat 1983 (3): 103-110

25 Thorpe SM, Poulsen HS, Pedersen KO, Rose C: Impact of standardization of estrogen and progesterone receptor assays of breast cancer biopsies in Denmark. Eur J Cancer Clin Oncol 1988 (24): 1263-1269

26 Haybittle JL, Blamey RW, Elston CW et al: A prognostic index in primary breast cancer. Br J Cancer 1982 (45):361-366

27 Todd JH, Dowle C, Williams MR, Elston CW, Ellis IO, Hinton CP, Blamey RW, Haybittle JL: Confirmation of a prognostic index in primary breast cancer. Br J Cancer 1987 (56): 489-492

The Contribution of Perturbed Epithelial-Mesenchymal Interactions to Cancer Pathogenesis

Seth L. Schor [1], Ana M. Schor [2], Anthony Howell [2], Ann Marie Grey [1], Martino Picardo [1], Ian Ellis [1] and Graham Rushton [2]

1 Department of Cell and Structural Biology, Stopford Building, University of Manchester, Manchester M13 9PL, United Kingdom
2 Cancer Research Fund, Department of Medical Oncology, Christie Hospital, Wilmslow Road, Manchester M20 9BX, United Kingdom

Interactions between epithelial cells and fibroblasts play a central role in directing both the spatial and temporal pattern of differentiation during the course of embryonic development [1]. Such "epithelial-mesenchymal" interactions continue to modulate and integrate various diverse elements of cell behaviour in the adult [2]. The biochemical identity of the signal molecules mediating epithelial-mesenchymal interactions has been the subject of intense investigation. Grobstein [3] first speculated that insoluble components of the extracellular matrix (ECM) might be involved; this initial insight has been confirmed in subsequent studies and there is now a substantial literature indicating that ubiquitous matrix macromolecules (such as collagens and proteoglycans) influence a variety of fundamental cellular attributes. The mechanism by which the ECM exerts these different effects appears to depend upon the interaction of matrix macromolecules with specific cell surface receptors resulting in alterations in the organisation of the cytoskeleton and consequent changes in cell shape [4].

Fibroblasts and epithelial cells also produce a number of soluble factors (cytokines) which function as paracrine regulators of cell behaviour [5]. Many of these appear to be members of "families" consisting of several structurally related isoforms. It is now apparent that cytokines are commonly multifunctional effectors capable of influencing such diverse aspects of cell behaviour as proliferation, migration and metabolic activity [6]; this complex spectrum of biological activity is modulated by the interplay of various parameters, including the concentration of free ligand [7], the presence of other cytokines in the cell milieu [8] and the precise class of receptor(s) present at the cell surface [9].

In the context of our understanding of the mediation of epithelial-mesenchymal interactions, it should be noted that the biological activity of both matrix macromolecules and cytokines are mutually interdependent in the sense that a) many cytokines exert a primary effect upon matrix biosynthesis by their respective target cells [10,11], b) the precise response of cells to cytokines may be determined by the nature of the ECM (by virtue of its consequent effect on cell shape) [13,14], and c) many cytokines bind with relatively high affinity to matrix molecules, in which bound form they may act directly on target cells or be released again as soluble agents upon degradation of the matrix [14]. The dynamic and reciprocal nature of these interactions between cells, matrix and cytokines allows for the generation of complex regulatory feedback loops which may act in either a negative (self-limiting) or positive (continuously amplifying) fashion.

Perturbations in normal cell-cell interactions have been postulated to contribute to the development of cancer [15], as well as other disease states characterised by abnormalities in epithelial proliferation and differentiation [16]. Such perturbations may result from a variety of causes, including the presence of aberrant fibroblasts producing inappropriate signalling cytokines and/or matrix macromolecules. We have previously reported that skin fibroblasts obtained from patients with breast cancer are aberrant (i.e., resemble foetal cells) in terms of their persistent production of an apparently novel cytokine, "migration stimulating factor" (MSF). In this chapter, we review our data concerning:

a) the identification, isolation and initial biochemical characterisation of MSF;
b) the mechanism of action of MSF on target cells;
c) the presence of MSF-secreting skin fibroblasts in breast cancer patients;
d) the potential involvement of MSF-secreting fibroblasts in cancer pathogenesis;
e) heterogeneity amongst fibroblasts in terms of MSF production, and
f) a "clonal modulation" model to account for the presence of MSF-secreting fibroblasts in cancer patients.

Identification, Isolation and Initial Characterisation of MSF

Fibroblasts plated onto the surface of 3D collagen gel substrata migrate down into the underlying macromolecular matrix at rates which are dependent upon a number of experimental parameters, including cell density [17]. Fibroblasts present within the collagen matrix are easily distinguished from those remaining on the gel surface and the percentage of such cells may be ascertained at any given time after plating by simple microscopic observation [18]. Using this experimental system, we reported that confluent foetal fibroblasts migrate into the 3D collagen matrix to a significantly greater extent than do their normal adult counterparts [17]. Initial studies concerned with the underlying biochemical basis of this observation indicated that incubation of adult cells with foetal fibroblast-conditioned medium results in a significant stimulation of cell migration [19]. These findings first led us to suggest that foetal fibroblasts produce a soluble "migration stimulating factor" (MSF). Related studies indicated that normal adult fibroblasts do not produce MSF, but retain responsiveness to it.

Foetal fibroblasts cultured *in vitro* undergo a spontaneous transition to a characteristically adult-like mode of migratory behaviour after 50-55 population doublings, i.e., approximately three-quarters of their *in vitro* life-span [17]. This acquisition of an adult migratory phenotype results from a concomitant cessation in MSF production [19].

The responsiveness of adult cells to MSF has provided the basis of a convenient bioassay for detecting its presence [19]. Briefly, this involves plating target adult fibroblasts onto 3D collagen gels at a confluent density (1-4 x 10^4 cells per m^2) in growth medium (MEM) containing 5% calf serum and the appropriate concentration of test material. The cultures are routinely incubated for 4 days and then fixed, stained and examined in an inverted microscope fitted with a photographic graticule defining a rectangular field. The number of cells present on the gel surface and within the underlying collagen matrix in 10-15 randomly selected microscopic fields are counted and this information is used to calculate the percentage of the total cell number present within the 3D collagen matrix. This bioassay has been employed to develop a purification protocol for MSF consisting of: a) an initial precipitation at 10% ammonium sulphate, b) heparin affinity chromatography (eluting at 0.3 M NaCl), c) FPLC gel filtration chromatography on a Superose-12 column, and d) FPLC reverse phase chromatography with a pro-RPC column [20]. The precipitation of MSF at such a low concentration of ammonium sulphate distinguishes it from the majority of other proteins in fibroblast conditioned medium and allows for an efficient initial purification.

MSF obtained by this protocol is cationic and yields a single band on SDS polyacrylamide gel electrophoresis with an apparent molecular mass of approximately 70 kDa. Our recent data indicate that there may be two molecular forms of MSF characterised by differences in N-terminal amino-acid sequence. These two species have provisionally been referred to as MSF-1 and MSF-2; further information regarding differences in their amino-acid sequence, biochemical properties and pattern of biological activity will be reported in a forthcoming publication (Grey et al., manuscript in preparation).

Cell migration into a 3D collagen matrix is clearly a complex biological endpoint which may be influenced by a variety of parameters. For example, initial studies designed to optimise the assay indicated that the extent of cell migration is dependent upon the particular batch of collagen used and the degree of confluency of target cells in the stock dish prior to trypsinisation [21]; these factors result in a certain degree of inter-experiment variation in the level of migration achieved in both control and MSF-stimulated cultures. Normal adult fibroblast lines characteristically display control levels of migration falling between 3-6%, compared to maximal MSF-stimulated levels of migration of 8-15%; within an individual experiment, MSF typically achieves a 3-5 fold relative stimulation of migration compared to the control. The level of reproducibility is good, with standard deviations for determinations made in replicate cultures generally less than 10% of the mean. We believe this assay system to have considerable advantages compared to others commonly used to measure migration (e.g., Boyden chambers), in that cell behaviour is assessed on a physiologically relevant substratum.

The Mechanism of Action of MSF on Target Fibroblasts

MSF has been characterised in a number of *in vitro* studies designed to elucidate the nature of its effect upon target cells and mechanisms of action. These have indicated that MSF displays a bell-shaped dose-dependent stimulation of cell migration, with maximal values achieved at concentrations between 1-10 ng/ml (Fig. 1) [22]. The molecular basis of this biphasic response to MSF is not understood and may reflect the involvement of distinctive classes of cell surface receptors (with different affinity constants).

Adult fibroblasts need not be continuously exposed to MSF during the 4-day incubation period of the bioassay in order for it to stimulate cell migration [22]. In this study, target adult fibroblasts growing in stock dishes were pre-incubated with MSF for varying periods of time prior to being trypsinised and then plated on the collagen gel substrata *in the absence of MSF*; pre-incubation for as little as 4-6 hours was found to be sufficient to give a maximal level of stimulation during the subsequent 4-day duration of the assay.

As discussed above, many cytokines appear to exert a direct effect upon matrix biosynthesis and/or degradation; these alterations in matrix turnover may then influence other fundamental aspects of cell behaviour, including migration. Our data suggest that MSF exerts a direct stimulatory effect upon the synthesis of a high molecular weight size class of hyaluronic acid (HA) and that production of this HA is required for the stimulation of cell migration [22].

HA (also known as hyaluronan) is a linear glycosaminoglycan consisting of repeated disaccharide subunits of glucuronic acid and N-acetylglucosamine. It is a major biosynthetic product of fibroblasts and has been shown to promote the migration of a number of cell types, including neural crest, cardiac cushion mesenchyme, corneal mesenchymal cells and fibroblasts. The involvement of HA in modulating cell migration *in vivo* has been particularly well documented during embryonic development; this biological function of HA appears to continue in the adult, with various lines of evidence implicating it in the regulation of cell movement in a number of pathological processes, such as wound healing and tumour invasion [23].

HA is a polydisperse macromolecule exhibiting significant variation in molecular mass in samples obtained from different tissue sources. The biological activity of HA has been shown to be critically dependent upon its size class in a number of experimental systems, including a) induction of angiogenesis [24], b) inhibition of cell proliferation [25], and c) induction of chondrogenic differentiation in chick embryonic mesenchymal cells [26]. Our data indicate that MSF stimulates the synthe-

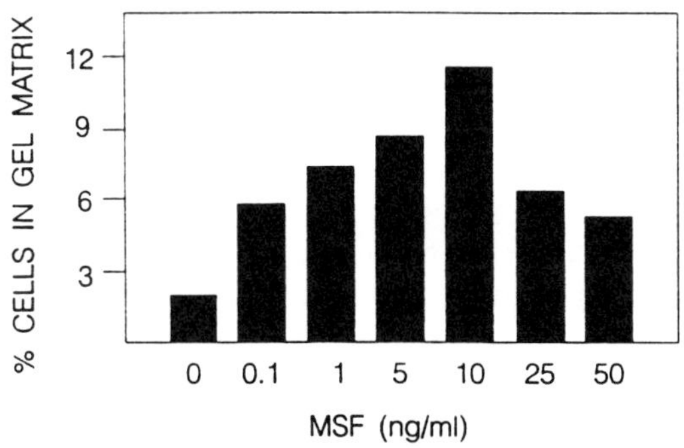

Fig. 1. The effect of different concentrations of MSF on the migration of a target adult fibroblast cell line

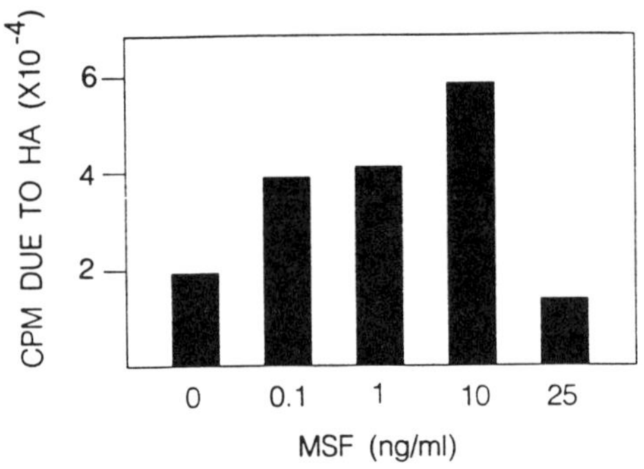

Fig. 2. The effect of different concentrations of MSF on the synthesis of hyaluronic acid by a target adult fibroblast cell line

sis of a high molecular weight size class of HA (i.e., >10^6 kDa) [22]. This stimulation reaches a maximum at 10 ng/ml MSF and declines back down to basal levels at higher concentrations (Fig. 2); this pattern of activity parallels the bell-shaped dose-response previously discussed with reference to migration and suggests a relationship between HA production and stimulation of migration. A more direct line of evidence is provided by observations that degradation of HA by exposure of target adult fibroblasts to *Streptomyces* hyaluronidase during the 4-day duration of the migration assay completely blocks the stimulation of cell migration by MSF; this suppression of MSF activity is observed both with fibroblasts continuously exposed to MSF during the migration assay, as well as for cells pre-incubated with MSF prior to plating on the collagen gels in the absence of any further MSF.

HA is synthesised by the enzyme hyaluronate synthase which is inserted in the plasma membrane. A detailed discussion of the factors which regulate its activity is beyond the scope of this review and may be found in several recent papers [27]. In the context of the present discussion, it should be noted that previous studies have indicated that the rate of HA synthesis in normal adult fibroblasts is critically dependent upon cell density, with significantly less HA being produced on a per cell basis in confluent cultures compared to subconfluent ones [28]. We have reported that the opposite is in fact the case for foetal fibroblasts, which display a relative increase in HA synthesis when cell confluence is achieved [29]. Our data suggest that the elevated level of HA synthesis by foetal cells at confluence may be due to its autocrine stimulation by MSF.

Previous studies have indicated that the biological activity of MSF is dependent upon the presence of serum (or plasma) in the growth medium [19]; it is for this reason that our standard bioassay is conducted in the presence of 5% calf serum. This dependence on serum clearly distinguishes MSF from certain other motility factors (such as autocrine motility factor) which are routinely assayed in serum-free medium [30]. The identity of the necessary constituent or constituents provided by serum have not been investigated.

The interaction of MSF with other well characterised cytokines has been examined. TGF-beta inhibits the intrinsically elevated level of migration displayed by foetal fibroblasts and blocks the stimulation of adult cell migration by MSF in a dose-dependent fashion (Fig. 3). This inhibitory effect of TGF-beta on the promotion of adult cell motility by MSF is accompanied by a parallel inhibition of the MSF-induced stimulation of HA biosynthesis; this observation is again consistent with the view that the stimulation of cell migration by MSF is in some fashion dependent upon an increase in HA production.

One further point needs to be emphasised. The ascription of a particular biological function to a cytokine (e.g., "migration stimulating factor") is generally a reflection of its activity in the bioassay used to measure it *in vitro* rather than a necessarily accurate description of its principal biological activity *in vivo*. In this regard, all the so-called "growth factors" have

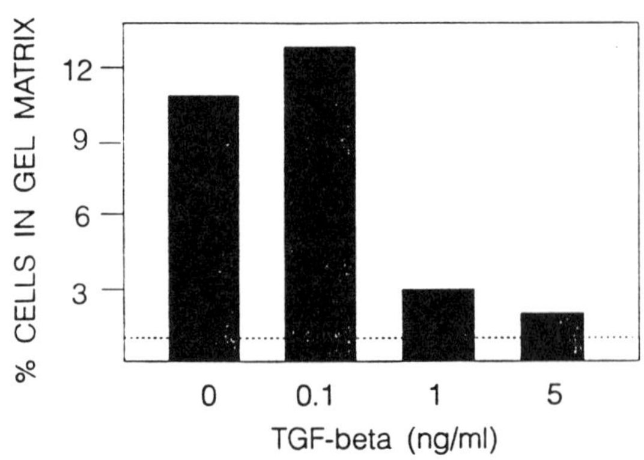

Fig. 3. TGF-beta prevents the stimulation of cell migration by MSF

well documented effects on various fundamental aspects of cell behaviour in addition to proliferation [6]. With this clear multifunctionality of cytokine action in mind, it should be noted that the principal biological activity of MSF *in vivo* may not relate to cell motility *per se*, but rather to some other aspect of cell function, such as HA production.

The Presence of MSF-Secreting Fibroblasts in Breast Cancer Patients

Much of our previous work has been concerned with documenting the presence of aberrant fibroblasts in breast cancer patients. These studies have demonstrated that a) tumour-derived fibroblasts obtained from approximately 50% of sporadic breast cancer patients expressed a foetal-like migratory phenotype [31,32], b) skin fibroblasts obtained from the same patients also exhibited foetal-like migratory behaviour, thus indicating the systemic nature of this stromal cell abnormality, and c) skin fibroblasts obtained from more than 90% of patients with familial breast cancer behaved in a similar foetal-like fashion [33]. The unaffected first-degree relatives of familial breast cancer patients are at a greatly elevated lifetime risk of developing breast cancer themselves [34]; it is therefore of interest that skin fibroblasts obtained from approximately 50% of such individuals displayed a foetal-like migratory phenotype [35]. This latter finding clearly indicates that the systemic presence of aberrant fibroblasts in individuals known to be at an elevated risk of developing breast cancer may precede the development of an overt malignancy.

Subsequent work has indicated that those cancer patient fibroblasts which display a foetal-like mode of migratory behaviour also differ from normal adult cells in terms of their continued production of MSF [19]. The MSF produced by cancer patient fibroblasts is indistinguishable from that made by foetal cells with respect to all of the biological and biochemical parameters that we have investigated to date. In contrast to the behaviour of foetal fibroblasts, the foetal-like fibroblasts of breast cancer patients do not undergo a spontaneous cessation in MSF production as a function of prolonged culture *in vitro* [36].

We have recently reported that detectable levels of MSF are present in the serum of breast cancer patients [37]. Serum was collected from two groups of patients. The first (untreated group) consisted of newly diagnosed patients (n=12) from whom serum was collected both 24 hours prior to surgical resection of the primary tumour mass and 4 days postoperatively; the second (treated) group consisted of patients (n=14) at various times after resection of the primary tumour (1-13 years) who had received or were receiving adjuvant therapy. Serum samples were also collected from age-matched healthy controls with no family history of breast cancer (n=20). Serum samples were fractionated by a simplified scheme involving a single gel filtration chromatography step and all fractions analysed for MSF in our standard bioassay; when present, migration stimulating activity was only observed in the expected fractions corresponding to a molecular mass of 60-70 kDa.

Our data indicate that MSF activity was present in 10/12 (83.3%) serum samples obtained from the untreated patients 24 hours prior to surgery and in 9/12 (75%) of these individuals 4 days following surgery (Fig. 4). It is important to note that the 5 negative samples in the pre- and postoperative group were obtained from different individuals; accordingly, 12/12 (100%) of the patients examined

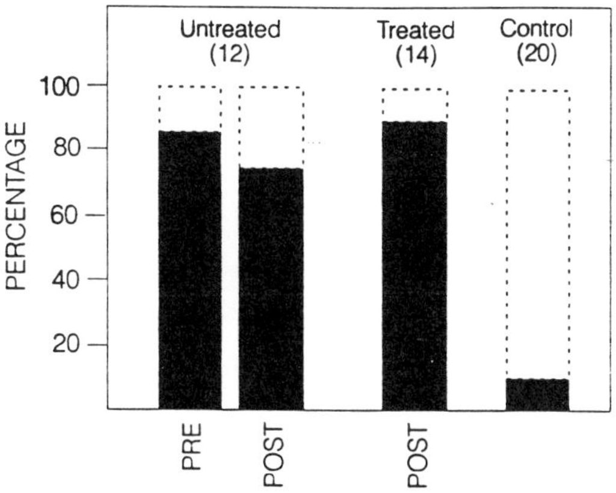

Fig. 4. The presence of MSF in the serum of breast cancer patients (untreated and treated) and healthy controls. Serum was obtained from the untreated patients both prior to (pre) and following (post) surgical resection of the primary tumour mass

were positive for MSF activity in at least one of the bioassays performed. Failure to detect MSF activity in the patient serum samples appears to reflect an occasional false negative in the assay, this generally being associated with a relatively high level of baseline migration in the assay control. Corresponding data obtained with the treated patients indicated the presence of detectable levels of MSF activity in 13/14 (93%) of the serum samples. Data obtained with the age-matched controls revealed the presence of MSF activity in only 2/20 (10%) of the samples. Biochemical characterisation of this activity indicated that is was indistinguishable from MSF produced by both foetal fibroblasts and the foetal-like fibroblasts of breast cancer patients.

The presence of MSF in the serum of the postoperative breast cancer patients in the absence of detectable residual disease clearly distinguishes MSF from previously described oncofoetal proteins, all of which are produced by the tumour itself and therefore act as indicators of tumour burden. Taken together with our results regarding the production of MSF by the skin fibroblasts of hereditary breast cancer patients and their unaffected first-degree relatives (discussed above), the observed presence of MSF activity in the serum of sporadic breast cancer cases appears to reflect the systemic presence of aberrant stromal fibroblasts in these individuals.

These findings have several potentially relevant clinical ramifications, one of them being the development of a novel screening regime for detecting individuals at elevated risk of developing breast cancer.

The Potential Involvement of MSF-Secreting Fibroblasts in Cancer Pathogenesis

On the basis of the above observations, we have put forward the following hypothesis suggesting a direct involvement of foetal-like fibroblasts in cancer pathogenesis [38]:

a) foetal fibroblasts undergo a programmed cessation in MSF production during the course of normal development which is manifest *in vitro* by the acquisition of an adult migratory phenotype;
b) this transition does not occur in certain individuals and,
c) the persistent production of MSF (as well as the possible expression of other aberrant phenotypic characteristics) by stromal fibroblasts in these individuals puts them at an elevated risk of developing cancer, most probably as a result of a dysfunction in normal epithelial-mesenchymal interactions.

Clonally derived subpopulations of foetal fibroblasts have been reported to undergo a spontaneous foetal-to-adult transition in migratory phenotype [17] and cessation in MSF production [19] as a function of *in vitro* ageing. It is conceivable that the persistent MSF-secreting fibroblasts present in cancer patients represent cells defective in the mechanism responsible for this transition and/or cells in which MSF synthesis has been reinitiated in response to some unidentified stimulus. The presence of MSF-secreting fibroblasts in cancer patients may also be accounted for by an alternative "clonal modulation" model of connective tissue function which will be discussed in the concluding section.

Experimental support of our suggestion that persistent foetal-like fibroblasts contribute directly to cancer pathogenesis has been provided by a number of independent studies. For example, Sakakura [39] observed that implantation of foetal (but not adult) fibroblasts in the adult rat mammary gland induced the hyperplastic growth of the normal epithelial elements and rendered these more sensitive to overt transformation by carcinogenic agents. In an immunolocalisation study using a monoclonal antibody capable of distinguishing foetal and adult fibroblasts, Bartal et al. [40] reported the presence of a subpopulation of positively staining (i.e., foetal-like) fibroblasts in the stroma associated with various types of tumour; their observation that not all of the tumour-associated fibroblasts stained positively is of particular relevance to our clonal modulation model.

There is a substantial literature documenting the presence of aberrant fibroblasts in patients with a variety of hereditary and apparently sporadic cancers of both epithelial and mesenchymal origin [38]; such cells have been reported to display a number of phenotypic characteristics commonly associated with transformation, such as colony formation in semi-solid medium and reduced serum requirement for growth. In the context of the present discussion, it should be noted that many of these transformation-associated behavioural characteristics are also features of normal foetal cells [41].

In the majority of previous studies dealing with the characterisation of cancer patient fibroblasts, the expression of aberrant phenotype characteristics by these cells has invariably been considered to reflect the existence of a systemic ("partially transforming") genetic lesion which only contributes to cancer development when expressed by the target epithelial cell population [42]. Our interpretation differs from this view in two fundamental respects, namely a) we consider the aberrant behaviour of the cancer patient skin fibroblasts to represent *persistent* foetal-like characteristics rather than the *acquisition* of a "partially transformed" phenotype, and b) we postulate a *direct* involvement of these foetal-like fibroblasts in disease pathogenesis. If this latter suggestion proves to be the case, it may be possible to design novel therapeutic agents targeted specifically at altering the behaviour of the aberrant fibroblast population (in contrast to the usual cytotoxic agents targeted at the cancer cells); such drugs might eventually make it possible to reduce the probability of developing cancer in identified high-risk individuals. In view of our data discussed in the previous section, TGF-beta may prove to be one such agent, being able to suppress MSF activity as well as inhibit epithelial and endothelial cell proliferation.

Cancer pathogenesis is generally regarded to be a multistep process involving an "initiating" genetic lesion followed by a series of subsequent events (collectively referred to as "progression"), these eventually leading to the clonal expansion of increasingly malignant cell populations [46]. In humans (as opposed to animal model systems), the process of progression may be quite indolent in nature and take many decades before malignant disease becomes apparent; indeed, it is not at all clear what proportion of aberrant (initiated) cell foci actually go on to form overt malignancies within the lifetime of the individual, although published reports suggest that this may not be very high [47]. According to our hypothesis, we suggest that perturbations in epithelial-mesenchymal interactions may result in a more permissive environment for the clonal expansion of such aberrant cells and contribute to the progressive development of a clinically recognised malignancy in this fashion. The MSF participating in such a sequence of events may originate from either neighbouring MSF-secreting fibroblasts or the systemic circulation (as indicated by the elevated levels of MSF in cancer patient serum).

Fibroblast Heterogeneity with Respect to MSF Production

Fibroblasts are a poorly defined group of cells which are identified *in vitro* on the basis of such non-specific parameters as spindle-shaped morphology, pattern of growth and the production of common matrix molecules, such as type I collagen. In spite of their similar appearance, it is now clear that fibroblasts actually represent a highly diverse cell population, with significant *inter-* and *intra*-site phenotypic heterogeneity [48]. Fibroblast subpopulations obtained from a given microregion of connective tissue have been demonstrated to differ in such fundamental properties as proliferative potential, matrix synthesis and cytokine production [49]. This heterogeneity has direct implications for tumour behaviour; for example, Dabbous et al. [50] have documented heterogeneity amongst fibroblasts in terms of their production of matrix-degrading enzymes in response to their interaction with carcinoma cells.

The possible existence of fibroblast heterogeneity with respect to MSF production has been investigated. An initial study involved characterising clonally-derived subpopulations of cells randomly selected from a parental foetal fibroblast line [17]. This work demonstrated the existence of a considerable degree of heterogeneity with respect to migratory phenotype, with a minority proportion of the subpopulations already behaving in a characteristically adult-like fashion. Twelve foetal-like subpopulations were followed for the duration of their *in vitro* life-span; 9/12 (75%) of these were observed to undergo a spontaneous transition to an adult-like mode of migratory behaviour and cease production of MSF (a characteristic of the parental line), whilst the remaining 3/12 (25%) continued to behave in a foetal-like fashion and produce MSF until senescence ensued. The potential significance of these findings to the behaviour of fibroblasts *in vivo* remains to be determined. One possibility is that they represent progenitors of persistently foetal-like cells in the adult (as detected in the breast cancer patients).

Ongoing studies in our laboratory have documented the presence of MSF-secreting fibroblasts in the normal adult. In the first of these, fibroblasts obtained from the skin and oral mucosa of 20 healthy controls were compared in terms of a number of parameters, including migratory phenotype and MSF production. Our data indicate that (as expected) fibroblasts obtained from the skin of only 2/20 (10%) of these individuals produced MSF; in contrast, fibroblasts obtained from 15/20 (75%) of the paired samples of oral mucosa were classified as foetal-like on the basis of their continued production of MSF. These data clearly demonstrate the existence of significant inter-site fibroblast heterogeneity with respect to MSF production.

A potential physiological function of MSF is suggested by its identification in 16/17 (94.1%) wound fluid samples examined [57]. Although the source of MSF in these samples is not known, it is possible that a subpopulation of adult dermal fibroblasts retains the capacity to resume the synthesis of MSF on a transient basis in response to tissue injury. The observed occurrence of directed fibroblast migration and elevated HA synthesis in wounds is consistent with a potential involvement of MSF in the wound healing response. It is also relevant in this context that wound healing in the oral mucosa is commonly recognised to differ from normal dermal healing in terms of both its speed and lack of extensive scar formation; it is possible that both of these advantageous features result from the presence of constitutive MSF-secreting fibroblasts in the oral mucosa.

The apparent involvement of MSF in wound healing may be particularly relevant to the view that tumours represent "wounds that do not heal" [43] and suggests that the same effects of MSF which contribute positively to normal wound healing when expressed locally and in a transient manner may promote cancer progression when they are systemic and/or prolonged in nature. Data indicating that MSF stimulates the synthesis of HA by target fibroblasts has been presented in the preceding section. Various studies have reported elevated levels of HA associated with the stroma of different types of tumour and provided evidence that this is correlated with more aggressive invasive behaviour [44]. HA has also been demonstrated to modulate a number of other processes of potential relevance to tumour development, including the proliferation of mammary epithelial cells [45] and angiogenesis [24].

Further data have revealed the existence of significant intra-site heterogeneity in fibroblasts derived from normal breast tissue [A.M. Schor et al., manuscript in preparation]; stromal cells obtained from the initial enzymatic digestion of the tissue (provisionally identified as *inter*-lobular fibroblasts) appear to constitutively produce MSF, whilst those stromal cells in close anatomical association with the epithelium (provisionally identified as *intra*-lobular fibroblasts) do not. In contrast to this situation in the normal breast, both intra and interlobular fibroblasts obtained from breast cancer patients appear to produce MSF and display a foetal-like mode of migratory behaviour.

A Clonal Modulation Model of Connective Tissue Function: Implications for the Presence of Foetal-Like Fibroblasts in Cancer Patients

As already mentioned, previous studies documenting the presence of aberrant fibroblasts in cancer patients have considered them to reflect the existence of an inherited genetic lesion which is present in all somatic cells, including fibroblasts. Such a "germ-line mutation" model may be applicable to the hereditary cancer syndromes, but cannot reasonably be invoked to explain the systemic presence of aberrant fibroblasts in patients with apparently sporadic forms of the disease.

We have proposed an alternative (but not necessarily mutually exclusive) "clonal modulation" model which we believe to be more consistent with the available experimental data [48]. According to this model, we suggest that a) there is a significant degree of both inter- and intra-site heterogeneity amongst fibroblasts with respect to MSF production (as well as other phenotypic characteristics), b) transient alterations in the relative proportion of specific fibroblast subsets may occur in response to pathological stimuli (e.g., wounding) and thereby play a role in the maintenance of tissue homeostasis, and c) persistent perturbations in the clonal balance of the fibroblast population are associated with the pathogenesis of various disease states characterised by a disruption of connective tissue function *per se* (e.g., scleroderma), as well as its interaction with epithelium (e.g., cancer). According to this epigenetic model, the MSF-secreting fibroblasts detected in cancer patients are not considered to be intrinsically aberrant cells, but rather an expanded subpopulation of cells also present in the normal adult. Numerous mechanisms might contribute to this postulated clonal expansion, including perturbed paracrine interactions with aberrant epithelial cell populations and/or exposure to environmental agents. An important corollary of the clonal modulation model is that the presence of "aberrant" fibroblasts in patients with hereditary cancer syndromes need not necessarily reflect the *expression* of the inherited genetic lesion in the fibroblasts themselves; expression of this lesion in other cell populations (perhaps of epithelial origin) could lead to the postulated clonal expansion of particular (e.g., MSF-producing) fibroblast subpopulations. In order to test this hypothesis we are currently investigating the extent of clonal heterogeneity in normal dermal fibroblasts in terms of MSF production and how the clonal balance of the population may be influenced by interaction with aberrant epithelial cell populations.

Finally, it must be emphasised that the clonal modulation model discussed here specifically addresses the question of the origin of the "aberrant" fibroblasts in cancer patients. It does not intrinsically conflict in any fashion with the multistep nature of carcinogenesis, nor does it diminish the well-documented genetic nature of the initiating step and continued major contribution of subsequent genetic lesions to progression events. The involvement of such genetic mechanisms (e.g., tumour suppressor genes) is unambiguous and need not be discussed in any detail. We do, however, wish to suggest that the data reviewed here underscores the importance of considering cancer as a disease in which many factors (not only genetic lesions) act in a concerted and complementary fashion to contribute to the ultimate clinical course of events. It should be remembered that genetic lesions may be present, but not necessarily expressed. Factors, such as cell-cell interactions, which contribute to the control of gene expression are therefore of fundamental importance. Evidence supporting this view has been provided by a number of earlier studies indicating that interactions of cancer cells with the host environment can repress expression of the malignant phenotype [51,52]. The importance of host factors in modulating expression of a malignant phenotype in epithelial cells transfected with oncogenes has been the subject of several recent communications [53,54]. In this latter study, Stoker et al. demonstrated that introduction of the v-src oncogene into chick embryo fibroblasts induced the expression of the expected range of transformation-associated phenotypic characteristics when the transfected cells were cultured *in vitro*; in spite of the fact that these cells were also tumourigenic when introduced into new-born chicks, their implantation into the developing embryo did not result in tumour development and lineage analysis indicated that the progeny of the transfected cells had contributed to various differentiated tissues.

Progress in the treatment of breast cancer (as well as other common forms of malignant disease) has been disappointingly slow as assessed by survival data. Zajicek [55,56] has commented on this point in editorial reviews and suggested that a broader appreciation of the factors contributing to cancer pathogenesis is required. We are in complete accord with this view and believe that a growing appreciation of the role played by cell-cell interactions in the control of gene expression promises to have significant end results in terms of devising improved means of patient management.

Summary

Foetal skin fibroblasts migrate into 3D collagen gels to a significantly greater extent than do adult cells. This enhanced motility of foetal fibroblasts appears to result from the production of a "migration stimulating factor" (MSF) which is not made by their normal adult counterparts. Adult skin fibroblasts retain responsiveness to MSF and cells exposed to this factor achieve the elevated levels of migration characteristic of foetal cells. MSF has been purified to homogeneity and characterised in terms of a number of biochemical criteria, including N-terminal amino-acid sequence. Studies concerned with the mechanism of action of MSF indicate that it stimulates the production of a high molecular weight class of hyaluronic acid (HA). Concurrent exposure of cells to *Streptomyces* hyaluronidase blocks the stimulation of adult fibroblast migration by MSF. In a related series of experiments, we have shown that TGF-beta inhibits the effects of MSF on both cell migration and HA production. Taken together, these data suggest that the stimulation of fibroblast migration by MSF is dependent upon (and may directly result from) a primary induction of HA synthesis.

We have previously reported that skin fibroblasts obtained from patients with sporadic and familial breast cancer, as well as the unaffected first-degree relatives of familial breast cancer patients, commonly display a foetal-like migratory phenotype. Subsequent work has indicated that a) these foetal-like cells also produce MSF, and b) detectable levels of MSF are present in the serum of sporadic breast cancer patients prior to and following surgical resection of the primary tumour mass. On the basis of these and related observations, we have put forward a hypothesis suggesting that the disruption in normal epithelial-mesenchymal interactions caused by the persistent production of MSF by fibroblasts in the adult may contribute directly to the pathogenesis of an epithelial cancer. The demonstration of aberrant fibroblasts in sporadic cancer patients (both in our own and independent studies) is not consistent with the "germ-line genetic lesion" model commonly invoked to account for the presence of such cells in patients with hereditary cancer syndromes. We have proposed an alternative "clonal modulation" in which we suggest that: a) a high degree of phenotypic diversity exists within fibroblast populations, b) a minority subpopulation of MSF-secreting fibroblasts is present in the normal adult, c) these cells may undergo a transient clonal expansion as part of tissue homeostatic mechanisms, such as wound healing, and d) the detection of MSF-secreting fibroblasts in cancer patients results from a persistent and inappropriate increase in their relative number in response to as yet unidentified stimuli; these may include interaction with emerging aberrant epithelial cell populations and/or environmental factors. Our recent data are consistent with this epigenetic model and indicate the existence of extensive inter- and intra-site heterogeneity amongst normal adult fibroblasts in terms of MSF production.

Acknowledgement

This work was supported by grants from the Cancer Research Campaign and Medical Research Council.

REFERENCES

1 Trelstad RL: Role of the Extracellular Matrix in Development. Academic Press, New York 1984
2 Cunha G, Bigsby RM, Cooke PS and Sugimura Y: Stromal-epithelial interactions in adult organs. Cell Differentiation 1985 (17):137-148
3 Grobstein C: Developmental role of the extracellular matrix. In: Slavkin H and Greulich RC (eds) Extracellular Matrix Influences on Gene Expression. Academic Press, New York 1975 pp 9-16
4 Hay ED and Svoboda KK: Extracellular matrix interactions with the cytoskeleton. In: Stein WD and Bronner F (eds) Cell Shape: Determinants, Regulation and Regulatory Role. Academic Press, San Diego 1989 pp 147-172
5 Sporn MB and Roberts AB: Peptide Growth Factors and Their Receptors (Vols I and II): Handbook of Experimental Pharmacology. Springer Verlag, Heidelberg 1990 Vol 95/1
6 Sporn MB and Roberts AB: Peptide growth factors are multifunctional. Nature 1988 (332):217-219
7 Cantrella M, McCarthy TL and Canalis E: Transforming growth factor-beta is a bifunctional regulator of replication and collagen synthesis in osteoblast-enriched cultures of fetal rat bone. J Biol Chem 1987 (262):2869-2874
8 Baird A and Durkin T: Inhibition of endothelial cell proliferation by type-beta transforming growth factor: interactions with acidic and basic fibroblast growth factors. Biochem Biophys Res Commun 1986 (138):476-482
9 Cheifetz S, Weatherbee JA, Tsang ML, Anderson JK, Mole JE, Lucas R and Massague J: The transforming growth factor-beta system: a complex pattern of cross-reactive ligands and receptors. Cell 1987 (48):409-415
10 Ignotz RA and Massague J: Transforming growth factor-beta stimulates the expression of fibronectin and collagen and their incorporation into the extracellular matrix. J Biol Chem 1986 (261):4337-4345
11 Balza E, Borsi L, Allemanni G and Zardi L: Transforming growth factor-beta regulates the levels of different fibronectingisoforms in normal cultured fibroblasts. FEBS Letters 1988 (228):42-44
12 Gospodarowicz D, Greenburg G and Birdwell CR: Determination of cellular shape by the extracellular matrix and its correlation with the control of cellular growth. Cancer Res 1978 (38):4155-4171
13 Colige A, Nusgens B and Lapiere CM: Effect of EGF on human skin fibroblasts is modulated by the extracellular matrix. Arch Dermatol Res 1988 (280 suppl):S42-S46
14 Rifkin DB and Moscatelli D: Recent developments in the cell biology of basic fibroblast growth factor. J Cell Biol 1989 (109):1-6
15 Rubin H: Cancer as a dynamic disorder. Cancer Res 1985 (45):2935-2942
16 Saiag P, Coulomb B, Lebreton C, Bell E and Dubertret L: Psoriatic fibroblasts induce hyperproliferation of normal keratinocytes in a skin equivalent model in vitro. Schience 1985 (230):669-672
17 Schor SL, Schor AM, Rushton G and Smith L: Adult, foetal and transformed fibroblasts display different migratory phenotypes on collagen gels: Evidence for an isoformic transition during foetal development. J Cell Sci 1985 (73):221-234
18 Schor SL: Cell proliferation and migration within three-dimensional collagen gels. J Cell Sci 1980 (41):159-175
19 Schor SL, Schor AM, Grey AM and Rushton GR: Foetal and cancer patient fibroblasts produce an autocrine migration-stimulating factor not made by normal adult cells. J Cell Sci 1988 (90):391-399
20 Grey AM, Schor AM, Rushton G, Ellis I and Schor SL: Purification of the migration stimulating factor produced by fetal and breast cancer patient fibroblasts. Proc Natl Acad Sci 1989 (86):2438-2442
21 Schor SL, Schor AM, Winn B and Rushton G: The use of three-dimensional collagen gels for the study of tumour cell invasion in vitro: experimental parameters influencing cell migration into the gel matrix. Int J Cancer 1982 (29):57-62
22 Schor SL, Schor AM, Grey AM, Chen J, Rushton G, Grant ME and Ellis I: Mechanism of action of the migration stimulating factor (MSF) produced by fetal and cancer patient fibroblasts: Effect on hyaluronic acid synthesis. In Vitro Cell Develop Biol 1989 (25):737-746
23 Knudson W, Biswas C, Li X-Q, Nemec RE and Toole BP: The role and regulation of tumor-associated hyaluronan. In: The Biology of Hyaluronan. Ciba Foundation Symposium 143. John Wiley and Sons, Chichester 1989 pp 150-159
24 Feinberg RN and Beebe DC: Hyaluronate in vascular genesis. Science 1983 (220):1177-1179
25 Goldberg R and Toole BP: Hyaluronate inhibition of cell proliferation. Arthritis Rheum 1987 (30):769-777
26 Kujawa MJ, Carrino DA and Caplan AI: Substrate-bonded hyaluronic acid exhibits a size-dependent stimulation of chondrogenic differentiation of stage 24 limb mesenchymal cells in culture. Dev Biol 1986 (114):519-528
27 Prehm P: Identification and regulation of the eukaryotic hyaluronate synthase. In: The Biology of Hyaluronan. Ciba Foundation Symposium 143. John Wiley and Sons, Chichester 1989 pp 21-31
28 Hronowski I and Anastassiades TP: The effect of cell density on net rates of glycosaminoglycan synthesis and secretion by cultured rat fibroblasts. J Biol Chem 1980 (255):10091-10099
29 Chen J, Grant M, Schor A and Schor SL: Differences between adult and foetal fibroblasts in the regulation of hyaluronate synthesis: correlation with migratory activity. J Cell Sci 1989 (94):577-589
30 Liotta L, Mandler R, Murano G, Katz DA, Gordon RK, Chiang PK and Schiffmann E: Tumor cell autocrine motility factor. Proc Natl Acad Sci 1986 (83):3302-3306
31 Durning P, Schor SL and Sellwood RAS: Fibroblasts from patients with breast cancer show abnormal migratory behaviour in vitro. Lancet 1984 (ii):890-892
32 Schor SL, Schor AM, Durning P and Rushton G: Skin fibroblasts obtained from cancer patients

display foetal-like migratory behaviour on collagen gels. J Cell Sci 1985 (73):235-244

33 Schor SL, Haggie J, Durning P, Howell A, Sellwood RAS and Crowther D: The occurrence of a foetal fibroblast phenotype in familial breast cancer. Int J Cancer 1986 (37):831-836

34 Ottman R, Pike MC, King M-C and Henderson BE: Practical guide for estimating risk in familial breast cancer. Lancet 1983 (ii):556-558

35 Haggie J, Schor SL, Howell A, Birch JM and Sellwood RAS: Fibroblasts from relatives of hereditary breast cancer patients display foetal-like behaviour in vitro. Lancet 1987 (i):1455-1457

36 Schor SL, Schor AM and Rushton G: Fibroblasts from cancer patients display a mixture of both foetal and adult-like phenotypic characteristics. J Cell Sci 1988 (90):401-407

37 Picardo M, Schor SL, Grey AM, Howell A, Laidlaw I, Redford J and Schor AM: The presence of migration stimulating activity in serum of breast cancer patients. Lancet 1990 (337):130-133

38 Schor SL, Schor AM, Howell A and Crowther D: Hypothesis: persistent expression of fetal phenotypic characteristics by fibroblasts is associated with an increased susceptibility to neoplastic disease. Exp Cell Biol 1987 (55):11-17

39 Sakakura T: Epithelial-mesenchymal interactions in mammary gland development and its perturbation in relation to tumourigenesis. In: Rich M, Hager J and Furmanski P (eds) Understanding Breast Cancer. Dekker, New York 1983 pp 261-284

40 Bartal AH, Lichtig C, Cardo CC, Feit C, Robinson E and Hirshaut Y: Monoclonal antibody defining fibroblasts appearing in fetal and neoplastic tissues. JNCI 1986 (76):415-419

41 Nakano S and Ts'O PO: Cellular differentiation and neoplasia: characterisation of subpopulations of cells that have neoplasia related growth properties in Syrian hamster embryo cell cultures. Proc Natl Acad Sci 1981 (78):4995-4999

42 Kopelovich L: Hereditary adenomatosis of the colon and rectum: relevance to cancer promotion and cancer control in humans. Cancer Gen Cytogen 1982 (95):333-351

43 Dvorak HF: Tumors - wounds that do not heal. N Engl J Med 1986 (315):1650-1659

44 Toole BP, Biswas C and Gross J: Hyaluronate and invasiveness of the rabbit V2 carcinoma. Proc Natl Acad Sci 1979 (76):6299-6303

45 Elstad CA and Hosick HL: Contribution of the extracellular matrix to growth properties of cells from a preneoplastic outgrowth: possible role of hyaluronic acid. Exp Cell Biol 1987 (55):313-321

46 Knudson AG: Genetics and etiology of cancer. In: Harris H and Hirschorn K (eds) Advances in Human Genetics. Raven Press, New York pp 1-66

47 Nielson M, Thomsen JL, Primdahl S, Dyreborg U and Anderson JA: Breast cancer and atypia among young and middle aged women. Br J Cancer 1987 (56):814-819

48 Schor SL and Schor AM: Clonal heterogeneity in fibroblast phenotype: implications for the control of epithelial-mesenchymal interactions. BioEssays 1987 (7):200-204

49 Hassell TM and Stanek EJ: Evidence that the healthy human gingiva contains functionally heterogeneous fibroblast subpopulations. Arch Oral Biol 1983 (28):617-625

50 Dabbous MK, Haney L, Carter LM, Paul AK and Reger J: Heterogeneity of fibroblast response in host-tumor cell-cell interactions in metastatic tumors. J Cell Biochem 1987 (35):333-344

51 Pierce GB: Differentiation of normal and malignant cells. Fed Proc 1970 (29):1248-1254

52 Mintz B and Illmensee K: Normal genetically mosaic mice produced from malignant teratocarcinoma cells. Proc Natl Acad Sci 1975 (72):3585-3589

53 Valverius EM, Ciardiello F, Heldin NE, Blondel B, Merlo G, Smith G, Stampfer MR, Lippman M, Dickson RB and Salomon DS: Stromal influences on transformation of human mammary epithelial cells overexpressing c-myc and SV40T. J Cell Physiol 1990 (145):217-216

54 Stoker AW, Hatier C and Bissell MJ: The embryonic environment strongly attenuates v-src oncogenesis in mesenchymal and epithelial tissues, but not in endothelia. J Cell Biol 1990 (111):217-228

55 Zajicek G: Progress against cancer: are we winning the war? Cancer J 1990 (3):2

56 Zajicek G: Clinical manifestations of transgenic cancer. Cancer J 1990 (3):3

57 Picardo M, Grey AM, McGurk M and Schor SL: Detection of migration stimulating activity in wound fluid. Exp Mol Pathol 1992 (in press)

Reporting Results from Adjuvant Therapy Trials with Special Emphasis on Quality-of-Life Findings

Richard D. Gelber [1], Monica Castiglione [2], Christoph Hürny [3], Jürg Bernhard [3], Alan Coates [3] and Aron Goldhirsch [4]

1 Harvard Medical School, Harvard School of Public Health, and Dana-Farber Cancer Institute, 44 Binney Street, Boston, MA 02115, U.S.A.
2 Institut für medizinische Onkologie, and International Breast Cancer Study Group Operation Office, Bern, Switzerland
3 International Breast Cancer Study Group Quality of Life Research Committee, Bern, Switzerland, and Sydney, Australia
4 Division of Oncology, Ospedale San Giovanni, Bellinzona, Ospedale Civico, Lugano, and Ospedale Beata Vergine, Mendrisio, Switzerland

Breast cancer is a major public health problem; it is estimated that more than 600,000 new patients will be diagnosed with invasive breast cancer in the world during 1991, more than 80 percent will have operable disease, and thus be candidates for adjuvant therapy. Less than 1% of these women, however, are anticipated to participate in randomised control clinical trials, making the data used to define appropriate treatments for all patients quite precious. Even modest treatment effects will influence the outcome for a large number of women. For node-negative disease, modest but important improvements in treatment efficacy may go undetected, and/or a much longer time may be required to identify an effective treatment.
Generally, in order to properly interpret results of clinical trials, it is required that some distinct aspects be considered: these include statistical uncertainty, relative magnitude of treatment effects, and absolute costs and benefits of treatment for a population. Exclusive emphasis on the p-value generates a misleading assessment of treatment effects, especially in subgroup analyses.
Furthermore, relying on the absolute difference in disease-free survival or overall survival curves at a single point underestimates the actual percent of patients who benefit.

Describing Treatment Benefit

What Do Life-Table Curves Show?

The main results from adjuvant therapy clinical trials are displayed in life-table curves such as those shown in Figure 1a from the NSABP Trial B-13 [1]. This trial was conducted on 679 patients with node-negative, oestrogen-receptor negative breast cancer. The figure shows the disease-free survival (DFS) comparison for patients treated with methotrexate-fluorouracil (M -> F) combination adjuvant chemotherapy for 13 months versus a surgery alone control group at 4 years median follow-up. The DFS curves show the percent of patients in each group who are estimated to remain disease-free at each time from randomisation. The results are often summarised by selecting one time (e.g., 4 years) and reporting the corresponding percent which remain disease-free for each group (e.g., 80% for treated patients and 71% for the surgical controls). However, at each time these curves divide the populations into proportions which: 1) remain disease free in the control group; 2) remain disease free in the treatment, but not in the control group, and 3) have an event even for the treated group. The percent of patients in each of

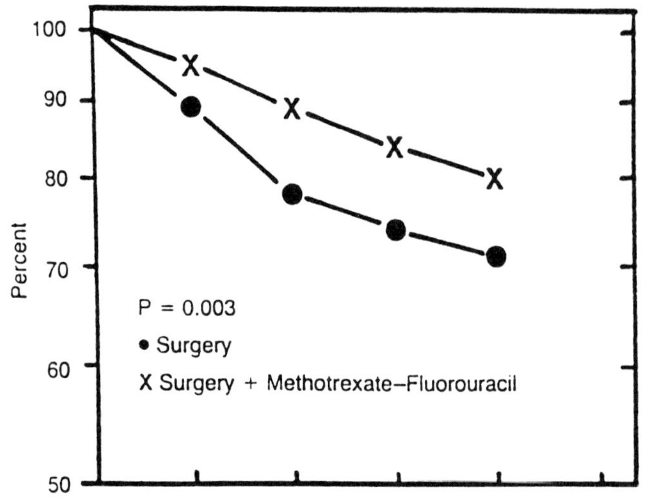

Year	0	1	2	3	4
No. at Risk •	340	258	171	111	62
No. at Risk X	339	268	190	112	58
Odds Ratio		2.20	2.18	1.93	1.81
P Value		0.009	0.0003	0.001	0.002

• 74 Events, X 44 Events

Fig. 1a. Disease-free survival according to treatment group among 679 patients with node-negative, oestrogen-receptor negative breast cancer in NSABP B-13 at 4 years median follow-up (reproduced with permission from ref. [1] p. 475)

these categories continually changes over time.

While some have argued that only the percent of patients between the 2 curves at a point in time benefit and all others do not, it is clear that this assessment which does not consider the time gained by treated patients compared to controls, is not particularly meaningful for patient decision making. In fact, it is possible that every patient in the treated group will have a longer disease-free survival time than if she had not received treatment. Specifically, a patient who is treated might have relapsed earlier if untreated, whether or not her relapse was destined to appear before or after 4 years. Thus, describing treatment benefit in terms of the absolute differences between DFS curves at a limited follow-up time point is an inadequate measure against which to weigh the

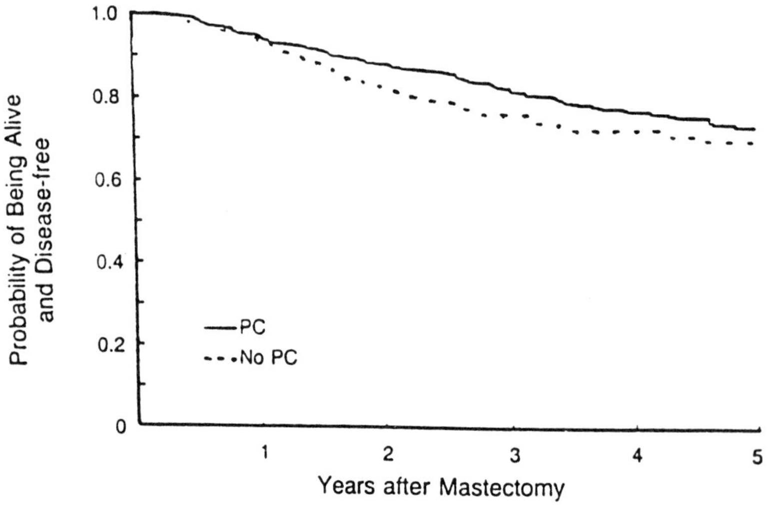

At Risk						
PC	848	801	668	447	273	98
No PC	427	400	318	205	126	53

Fig. 1b. Disease-free survival according to treatment group among 1275 patients with node-negative breast cancer in International (Ludwig) Trial V at 42 months median follow-up (reproduced with permission from ref. [2] p. 492). Note: PC denotes perioperative chemotherapy

costs of treatment. Figure 1a also illustrates that despite an improved outcome for the treated group, a large proportion of patients are estimated to relapse even if treated. This identifies the magnitude of additional potential gains for more effective treatments.

The impression provided by the life-table curve regarding the magnitude of the treatment effect is related to the way the curves are displayed. Figure 1b shows the disease-free survival curves for perioperative chemotherapy (PC) and for no adjuvant therapy (No PC) from the International (Ludwig) Trial V at 42 months median follow-up published simultaneously with the NSABP Trial B-13 [2]. The effectiveness of the PC as illustrated in Figure 1b appears to be much less than the effectiveness of M -> F as illustrated in Figure 1a. However, the DFS curves for NSABP B-13 are more boldly drawn, have a vertical axis which is truncated at 50%, and are plotted on a logarithm scale. (Note that truncating the scale focuses attention on the proportion of the population for which treatment effects might be demonstrated, and plotting the curves on a logarithm scale gives the slopes of the straight lines an interpretation as the yearly risk of an event.)

Figure 1c shows the International Trial V DFS curves based on the 42-month median follow-up data [2] plotted in the style similar to that of the NSABP B-13 results. The effectiveness of the perioperative chemotherapy course given to patients in this trial now appears to be larger than it first appeared from Figure 1b. Statistically significant p-values are shown in both Figures 1a and 1c, and the redrawing of the life-table curves increases our confidence that both the International Trial and NSABP B-13 demonstrate that adjuvant chemotherapy is effective for patients with node-negative breast cancer. In fact, the effectiveness of the single course of perioperative chemotherapy is estimated to be about half that of the 13-month chemotherapy regimen (22 percent reduction in the relative risk of an event compared with 45 percent, respectively). Four-year DFS percentages for the control and treated groups were 71% and 80% for B-13, and 73% and 77% for Trial V [1,2]. The p-values reflecting the statistical uncertainty of these observed differences were 0.003 and 0.04, respectively, and were based upon 118 events in B-13, and 276

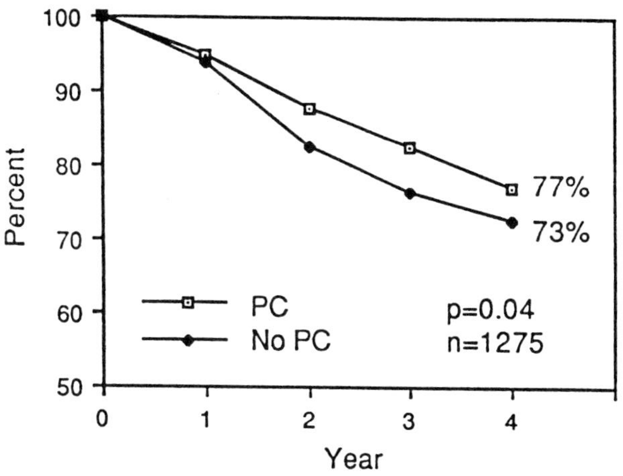

Fig. 1c. Disease-free survival according to treatment group among 1275 patients with node-negative breast cancer in International (Ludwig) Trial V at 42 months median follow-up: results from Figure 1b displayed according to the style of Figure 1a

events in Trial V. Fewer events were needed in the first study because the observed treatment difference was larger.

What Does the P-Value Measure ?

Quite often the single (or at least most prominent) statistic that accompanies the presentation of life-table curves is the p-value (probability value) for the observed difference. This value is frequently incorrectly used as a measure of the magnitude of the true treatment effect. If the p-value is less than or equal to 0.05, we declare with joy that the treatment is effective; if, however, the p-value is greater than 0.05, we declare that the treatment has no effect. This inappropriate interpretation of the p-value as a measure of treatment effect ($p \leq 0.05$ indicating an effective treatment, while $p > 0.05$ indicating a completely ineffective treatment) creates unnecessary controversy and confusion both for the overall evaluation of clinical trial results and especially for analyses within subgroups of patients.

The p-value is a measure of the statistical uncertainty of an observed result, and depends not only on the magnitude of the treatment effect, but also on the number of events that have been observed for the statistical analysis. Technically, the p-value is the probability of obtaining the observed treatment effect difference (or one more extreme) if we assume that the true treatment effects are identical (i.e., assuming the null hypothesis). In other words, given the number of events that have been observed in the treatment and control groups, the p-value indicates how likely it was to have observed the given study outcome differences by chance alone. If the p-value is small (e.g., a less than 5% chance that the more extreme differences could happen by chance alone), we traditionally accept this as evidence that the observed treatment differences are real (i.e., not likely due exclusively to the play of chance).

Unfortunately, some have also adopted the opposite tradition of claiming that if the p-value is greater than 0.05, then the entire observed difference must be due to the play of chance, and in fact, there is no evidence indicating a treatment effect. The fallacy of such an interpretation is illustrated by the results in Figure 2. Disease-free survival curves are shown for treated and control groups having exactly the same treatment effect as that observed for the International Trial V at 42 months median follow-up (Fig. 1c), but with half the number of patients and half the number of events as the actual Trial V. With half the number of events, the observed treatment difference is no longer statistically significant (p=0.16), and some would therefore report

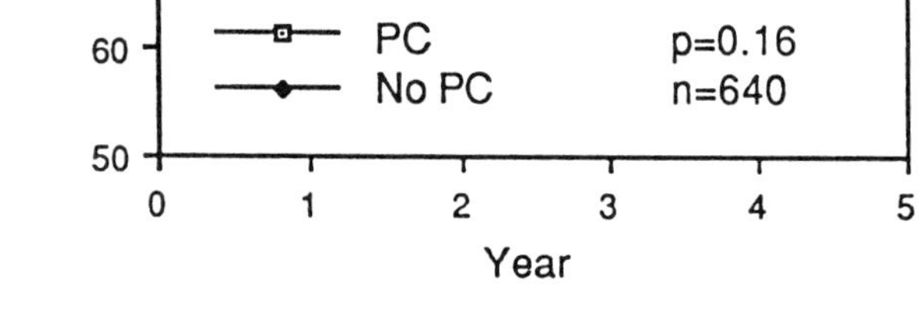

Fig. 2. Disease-free survival according to treatment group assuming an identical outcome as International Trial V at 42 months median follow-up, but for one-half the number of patients entered (and one-half the events observed)

that perioperative chemotherapy has no effect. Figure 2 and Figure 1c differ only with respect to the number of patients and events that contribute to the observed results. And yet, based on the p-value some interpret Figure 1c as demonstrating a treatment effect, while Figure 2 demonstrates no therapeutic relevance. Given that the curves in the 2 figures are exactly the same, there is obviously something wrong with the above interpretation.

What Are Relative and Absolute Measures of Treatment Effect ?

In order to illustrate 2 useful measures of treatment effect, the disease-free survival curves at 5-years' median follow-up for International Trial V are presented in Figure 3. An *absolute measure of treatment effect* is the difference between the disease-free survival curves at 5 years, 6% with standard error of ± 3% in this example. A *relative measure of treatment effect* is the ratio of the risk (or hazard) of an event in the treated group relative to the risk of an event in the control group (known as the hazard ratio). In this example, the hazard ratio is 0.78 with 95% confidence interval (0.63 to 0.96). This indicates a 22% reduction in the risk of relapse for treatment compared with control.

Some prefer the absolute measure because it appears to reflect more accurately the treatment effect for all patients. However, the magnitude of the estimates derived in this way depends on which time point is chosen. For example, based on Figure 3, at 1 year the difference is 1% in favour of treatment, while at 2 years it is 5%, at 3 years it is 7%, and at 5 years it is 6%. Is it then correct to say that only 6% of patients benefit and therefore 94% gain nothing from treatment? Furthermore, this estimate of the "percent of patients who benefit" ignores the fact that treatment effects influence different portions of the population over time. Specifically, based on the control group in Trial V (Fig. 3), 17% of the patients have the potential to benefit within 3 years (i.e., 3-year DFS is 83%), 32% have the potential to benefit within 5 years, and an increasing percent of patients are candidates for benefit beyond 5 years. The absolute measure of treatment effect at any time is constrained to be

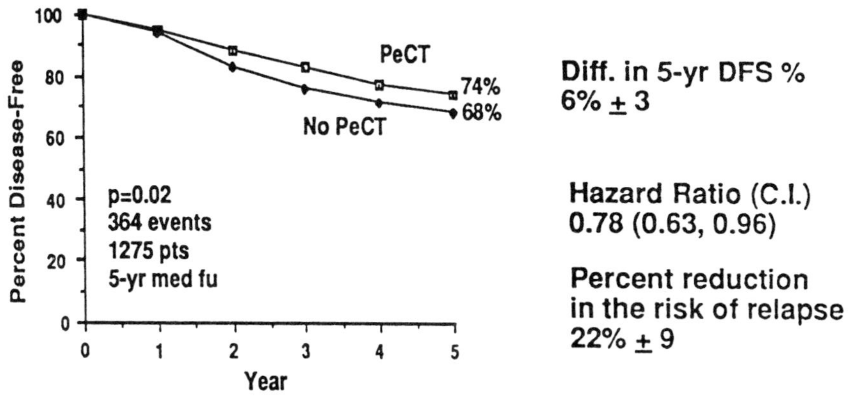

Fig. 3. Disease-free survival according to treatment group among 1275 patients with node-negative breast cancer in International Trial V at 5 years median follow-up: relative versus absolute measures of treatment effect. PeCT denotes perioperative chemotherapy

less than the estimated proportion of patients in the control group who would have an event up to that time. Thus, at five years a completely 100% effective treatment in International Trial V could produce a maximum absolute treatment effect of 32%. Furthermore, the importance of a given absolute treatment effect (of 6%, say), as well as the possibility to detect the effect, depends on the baseline prognosis of the control group. An improvement from 92% to 98% DFS represents a qualitatively different advance than one from 26% to 32% DFS.

Relative measures estimate the effect of treatment at reducing the risk of an event compared with the control group. Relative measures have the advantage that they can be used to compare treatment effects across subgroups of patients which have different baseline prognoses, and should be included more often in trial reports.

Are There Alternative Ways to Express Treatment Benefit ?

None of the previously described alternatives (either absolute risk reduction or relative risk reduction) adequately considers the aspect of time. The average time gained for the population of treated patients compared with the control patients is estimated by the area between the disease-free survival curves for these 2 groups [3,4]. For example, Figure 4 shows the average number of disease-free survival months gained by perioperative chemotherapy as compared with no perioperative chemotherapy as a function of the time from entry into the International Trial V. This average gain is obtained by calculating the area between the disease-free survival curves shown in Figure 3. It is interesting to note that the gain for the treated patients increases as the time from study entry increases. Thus, relatively small early gains in average months of disease-free survival, such as those illustrated in Figure 4, represent a small percentage of the potential gains that might be achieved with additional follow-up, since the disease-free survival curves are likely to remain separated in the future.

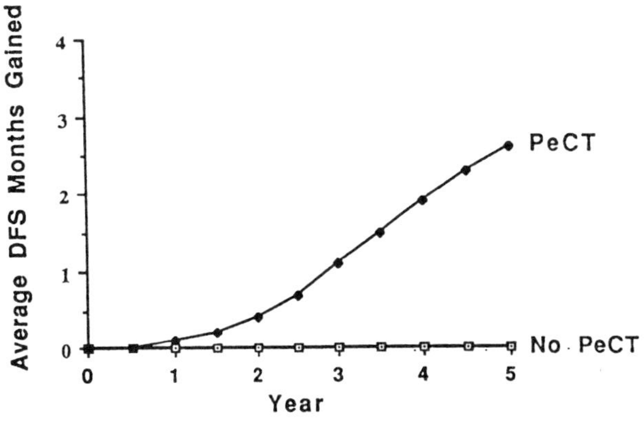

Fig. 4. Average months of disease-free survival (DFS) gained for the perioperative chemotherapy group compared with the no adjuvant treatment group in International Trial V through the first 5 years of follow-up. PeCT denotes perioperative chemotherapy.

Subgroup Analyses

Are Subgroup Analyses Really Forbidden ?

Subgroup analyses are performed to determine whether treatment effects are similar for different groups and across studies. Their conduct often produces controversy and some argue that their usefulness is less than their ambiguity. We believe that the difficulty associated with subgroup analysis is primarily related to the overinterpretation of the attached p-value. The p-values associated with these analyses no longer provide an accurate measure of the probability that the observed outcomes would happen by chance alone [5]. Also, because the number of events will vary from subgroup to subgroup due to sample size and hazard rate differences between subgroups, misusing the p-values as measures of treatment effect (incorrectly taking $p \leq 0.05$ to indicate a treatment effect, while $p > 0.05$ indicates no treatment effect) creates controversy and promotes misleading conclusions about treatment recommendations. Multiple subgroup analyses lead to an increased chance of a false-positive result. For example, if 10 independent subgroups are evaluated for treatment effects, the chance of observing at least one $p \leq 0.05$ is 40%. In addition, apparent treatment effect-patient subgroup interactions are quite likely to appear by chance alone [5]. If an overall treatment comparison reaches statistical significance (p=0.05) and we divide the population into 2 randomly selected halves, there is a one-third chance that all of a statistically significant result will appear in one-half of the population (p=0.03), while the other half will exhibit a non-significant result (p=0.48).

Subgroup analyses are done to determine if patient sub-populations have a different degree of responsiveness to a given treatment (i.e., lower versus higher relative reduction in the risk of an event under treatment). This is different from the search for prognostic factors which define patient subpopulations which have different baseline risks for an event. These 2 separate aspects, baseline prognosis and treatment responsiveness, are often confused when the concept of prognostic factors is discussed. Furthermore, if the database used in a search for prognostic factors includes treated patients, then the

Table 1. Distinction between a prognostic factor and a treatment responsiveness factor

A: PROGNOSTIC FACTOR: Nodal status in the overview of tamoxifen trials

Nodal status	5-year mortality percents: Control	Tamoxifen	Difference	Percent mortality reduction ± s.d.
N0/N-	18%	15%	3%	15% ± 8
N 1-3	25%	20%	5%	17% ± 8
N 4+	48%	41%	7%	17% ± 6
All Patients	32%	27%	5%	18% ± 3

B: TREATMENT RESPONSIVENESS FACTOR: Oestrogen receptor (ER) status in International (Ludwig) Trials III and IV for postmenopausal node-positive patients

ER status	7-year event* percents: Observation	Prednisone & tamoxifen	Difference	Percent event reduction ± s.d.
ER+ (≥10 fmol)	77%	64%	13%	30% ± 14
ER - (0-9 fmol)	79%	81%	-2%	-19% ± 25
Both (ER+, ER-)	78%	70%	8%	15% ± 13

* Event: relapse, second malignancy or death, whichever occurs first

prognostic significance of treatment responsiveness factors will be exaggerated (e.g., oestrogen receptor status for patients receiving endocrine therapy). Table 1 illustrates the distinction between a *prognostic factor* and a *treatment responsiveness factor*. In the analysis of mortality in the tamoxifen overview [6,7], nodal status was found to be a prognostic factor as indicated by the increasing mortality percents for the control group. However, nodal status in this analysis was not a treatment responsiveness factor as the treatment effects estimated by the percent mortality reduction were similar across all nodal groups.
In contrast, oestrogen receptor (ER) status in the 7-year analysis of International (Ludwig) Trials III and IV for postmenopausal node-positive patients [8] was not a prognostic factor as indicated by the similar outcomes for the observation groups. However, one year of tamoxifen and low-dose prednisone was more effective at reducing the risk of events for patients in the ER+ than in the ER- cohort, illustrating that ER status was a treatment responsiveness factor in this study. Consequently, ER status was a significant prognostic factor for patients who received this endocrine therapy (64% vs. 80% event percents for ER+ vs. ER- subgroups, respectively) compared with those in the observation group (77% vs. 79%).

Meta-Analysis (Overview)

Are the Answers Obtained Always Useful?

We discussed the method of meta-analysis in previous issues of this Monograph. The meta-analysis conducted in 1985 of all randomised trials investigating adjuvant systemic therapy for breast cancer with either tamoxifen or chemotherapy [6,7] is distinguished from other procedures for combining results by using the label "overview". A proper overview is conducted according to several principles designed to avoid introducing systematic biases into the analysis. An overview analysis includes randomised trials which compare 2 groups of patients who receive identical therapies, except that the study treatment is included for one group but not for the other. Treatment effects are estimated by comparing like with like within each trial before the results are combined across all studies; only properly randomised trials are included; all relevant trials are included; and all patients are included as randomised.
The purpose of a meta-analysis for investigating adjuvant therapies for breast cancer is to increase the number of events available to test the null hypothesis of no treatment effect. Individual studies are often too small to provide sufficient evidence to detect modest but humanly worthwhile treatment differences. Increasing the number of events improves the statistical precision of the results and enables detection of smaller differences. The meta-analysis also facilitates the evaluation of treatment effect separately within relevant subgroups of the patient population. Because the null hypothesis assumes no treatment effect for each of the studies being combined, there is no requirement that the trials be very similar in order to assure the validity of the analysis. The overview is, therefore, extremely useful as a guide to determine whether a series of "negative" results from individual trials truly indicates the absence of any treatment effect, or is a consequence of too few events in the separate studies.
Interpretation of the treatment effect estimates requires an appreciation of indirect comparisons and the use of the arithmetic construction [9]. The magnitudes of treatment effects estimated by 2 separate meta-analyses may not be directly comparable due to differences in patient or study selection that contributed to the separate analyses. Such indirect comparisons are not protected by the principle of comparing like with like, and must therefore be validated by results from direct comparisons within randomised clinical trials.
The breast cancer overview evaluating tamoxifen included trials of tamoxifen vs. no adjuvant treatment (nil), and trials of tamoxifen plus other therapy vs. the same other therapy (arithmetic construction) [9]. The results for 3,600 patients under the age of 50 are shown in Table 2. No mortality reduction was observed for the treated patients (estimated percent reduction in odds of death ± s.e. = -1% ± 8%). However, over three-quarters of the information was derived from studies in which tamoxifen was combined with chemotherapy.

Table 2. Arithmetic construction: Tamoxifen overview for age < 50

	Percent reduction (± s.e.) in odds of:	
	Recurrence	Death
All Trials	16% ± 6	-1% ± 8
Tamoxifen versus no adjuvant treatment	32% ±10	21% ±14
Tamoxifen and chemotherapy versus same chemotherapy	8% ± 7	-9% ± 9

from Early Breast Cancer Trialists' Collaborative Group [7]

The percent reduction in the odds of death was -9% ± 9% for the trials of tamoxifen plus chemotherapy versus chemotherapy, while it was 21% ± 14% for the trials of tamoxifen versus no adjuvant treatment. Thus, more recent individual trials which indicate positive effects of tamoxifen for younger node-negative patients with ER-positive tumours are not inconsistent with the overview results when the component parts of the arithmetic construction are critically examined.

Integrating Quality of Life Information

Can Quality of Life be Measured?

Quality of life of breast cancer patients receiving systemic therapy has been studied in advanced disease when treatments are applied with palliative intent [10-12]. In the adjuvant setting, however, therapies associated with acute toxic effects are administered during a time when patients are free of disease-related symptoms. The expectation is that the investment of this period of toxicity will be balanced by the delay in relapse and improvement in survival for the future. The toxic effects are felt by the entire population of patients, while it is possible that the benefits of treatment might be enjoyed only by some.

Quality of life is a multidimensional and subjective entity which is impossible to measure in absolute quantitative terms. It is influenced by all aspects of life including health, psychosocial well-being, and the subjective sense of satisfaction. Measurement of treatment effects on quality of life might be more feasible. First attempts at assessing the impact of treatments on quality of life were made by identifying and grading the side effects of treatment. Subsequent efforts have been made to measure patients' perceptions of the influence of side effects of adjuvant treatment, and patients' perceptions of symptoms of disease and treatment for relapse.

Several instruments have been developed to assess quality of life and these have been reviewed for their attributes and value for eliciting patient perceptions which are reliable and responsive to treatment differences. Recent reviews by Maguire and Selby [13], Donovan et al. [14] and Moinpoir et al. [15] discuss some of the instruments that have been used for cancer patients. Levine et al. [16] have developed an interviewer-administered questionnaire specifically designed to evaluate the quality of life of breast cancer patients who receive adjuvant chemotherapy. The Breast Cancer Chemotherapy Questionnaire (BCQ) consists of 30 items administered in a 15-minute interview. The items investigate 7 areas of assessment including loss of attractiveness, fatigue, physical symptoms, inconvenience, emotional distress, feelings of hope, and support from others. The questionnaire was applied to evaluate quality of life in a randomised study that compared 2 different durations of adjuvant chemotherapy (12 weeks vs. 36 weeks). The results of the quality-of-life assessment indicate a more rapid improvement in the mean BCQ score following completion of the 12-week course with a reduced score continuing for patients treated with the 36-week regimen. The BCQ was able to distinguish those patients receiving adjuvant chemotherapy beyond 12 weeks from those who had completed it, thus providing a numerical value associated with the administration and completion of chemotherapy [17].

In 1986 through 1989, the International Breast Cancer Study Group (IBCSG) initiated Trials VI through IX to investigate adjuvant treatments for women with operable breast cancer. The studies are designed to evaluate the duration and timing of chemotherapy and endocrine therapy for premenopausal patients (Trials VI and VIII), and the use, duration, and timing of chemotherapy added to tamoxifen for postmenopausal patients (Trials VII and IX). The anticipated subjective side effects in the various randomly assigned treatment options are very different, and therefore, aspects of quality of life are being assessed. Because the trials are being conducted in 20 centres in 9 different countries worldwide, the measurement instrument had to be practical, able to be completed with a minimum of professional supervision, and applicable in 11 different languages. The Group's objective is to achieve a high degree of compliance, and to make quality-of-life issues routinely considered for treatment comparisons.

The 2-page questionnaire adopted by the IBCSG consists of 5 scales designed to obtain a patient's perceptions on different aspects of her quality of life (Fig. 5). Three linear analogue self-assessment (LASA) scales are included for physical well-being, mood, and appetite. Each scale is presented as a 10-centimeter line with a descriptive adjective written at each of the extremes. Physical well-being ranges between good and lousy, mood ranges between happy and miserable, and appetite ranges between good and none. The patient is asked to place a mark along the line to describe her current condition. Visual analogue scales are widely used in other aspects of psychological measurement [18], and there is precedent for their use in breast cancer trials to which they were first applied by Priestman and Baum [11]. These authors used a series of 10 linear-analogue self-assessment scales to monitor subjective benefits of treatment, and later expanded the instrument to compare alternative treatments for breast cancer [19]. Coates et al. [20] investigated a subset of these LASA scales in patients with melanoma, lung cancer and ovarian cancer. They found that the LASA methodology was practical and feasible, and that the association between LASA scores and known factors such as performance status and response category provided evidence of the validity of the technique [20,21].

The fourth item on the IBCSG questionnaire (Fig. 5) is the Personal Adjustment to Chronic Illness Scale (PACIS), also known as the subjective life change unit score (SLCU), a one-item self-assessment instrument developed by Rahe [22]. The patient answers the question, "How much effort does it cost you to cope with your illness?" by marking a scale from 0 (no effort at all) to 100 (a great deal). The scale has been used with good compliance in the Swiss subset of patients of International Trial V and several other studies with cancer patients [23-26]. Rogentine et al. [27] found in a prospective study of melanoma patients that the amount of adjustment needed to cope with this illness (as measured by the SLCU) was an important prognostic factor in predicting 1-year disease-free survival after operation.

The fifth instrument in the IBCSG questionnaire is the Bf-S (Befindlichkeits-Skala) [28,29], a 28-item adjective checklist with a dichotomous response format designed for unidimensional (one main factor) assessment of well-being/mood with high sensitivity for depression (Fig. 5). It is shorter and less burdensome for the patient than the Profile of Mood States (POMS) multidimensional scale, and is therefore more likely to have transcultural stability of factor structure and is less likely to be biased by language differences.

The self-administered questionnaire is presented to the patient prior to beginning any therapy, 2 months after starting therapy, and every 3 months for 2 years. When the patient relapses, 2 additional assessments are done, one within one month, and the other at 6 months post-relapse.

Preliminary results are now available for 2093 patients randomised in the trials. As an example of results the sequential pairwise analysis of scores provided by the Personal Adjustment to Chronic Illness Scale (PACIS) for postmenopausal patients (Trials VII and IX) is shown in Figure 6. Square roots of the score are shown and used in the analysis in order to obtain more normally distributed results. The sequential pairwise analysis illustrates changes in score from one time point to the next time point based only on patients who have reports at both assessments. This adjusts for patient cohort differences over time. Lower scores indicate less effort of the patients to cope with their disease (i.e., improved adjustment).

Individual scores range from 0 (no effort at all to cope) to 100 (a great deal of effort to cope). Trials VII and IX are still accruing patients, so 647 postmenopausal patients provide coping scores for both of the first 2 assessments, and leave blank

page 1 of 2

INTERNATIONAL BREAST CANCER TRIALS
STUDY VI AND VII QUALITY OF LIFE FORM (FORM QL)

INSTRUCTIONS: The patient is asked to fill in this questionnaire within four weeks of operation and every three months over two years, in the clinic (before getting chemotherapy, if any).

☐ Language

Patient's Name ______________ Clinic's Name ______________

☐☐ Bf-S (from pg 2)

Randomization number ☐☐☐☐☐ Clinic sequence number ______

☐☐ ☐☐ ☐☐ Date this form completed (day,month,year)

Please spare a moment to answer the following questions. Your information will be treated as strictly confidential. Thank you for replying!

Please mark a cross (X) according to how you rate the following aspects overall, for the entire period since your last full clinical assessment.

> Example—
> TIREDNESS:
> None ——————————X—————— A lot
>
> This would indicate considerable tiredness since your last assessment.

☐☐☐ PHYSICAL WELL-BEING:
Good ______________________ Lousy

☐☐☐ MOOD:
Happy ______________________ Miserable

☐☐☐ APPETITE:
Good ______________________ None

Please answer the following question by putting a cross (X) between 0 and 100 according to your self-evaluation.

How much effort does it cost you to cope with your illness?

☐☐☐ no effort at all |—|—|—|—|—|—|—|—|—|—| a great deal
0 20 40 60 80 100

Fig. 5. International Breast Cancer Study Group quality-of-life questionnaire for Trials VI, VII, VIII and IX. The form is completed by the patient at the start of treatment, 2 months later, and every 3 months thereafter for 2 years. It is also completed 1 month and 6 months following relapse.

INTERNATIONAL BREAST CANCER TRIALS
STUDY VI AND VII QUALITY OF LIFE FORM (FORM QL)

Patient's Name ______________________________ Clinic's Name ________________

Randomization number ________________________ Clinic sequence number______

Below you will find different words. Please decide -- without thinking too much -- which of the two corresponds most closely to your present state or the way you feel now. Put a cross in the box to the left of this word. Only if you are completely unable to make a decision, mark the box in the column "neither/nor." Do not skip any line!

I am feeling now:

	more		more		neither/nor
1.		alert		listless	
2.		reserved		responsive	
3.		cheerful		downcast and blue	
4.		successful		unsuccessful	
5.		irritable		calm	
6.		indecisive		decisive	
7.		joyful		tearful	
8.		good-humoured		ill-humoured	
9.		lazy		active	
10.		sociable		withdrawn	
11.		worthless		of full value	
12.		relaxed		tense	
13.		happy		unhappy	
14.		shy		bold	
15.		desperate		hopeful	
16.		secure		threatened	
17.		abandoned		cared for	
18.		well-balanced		unbalanced	
19.		confident		insecure	
20.		miserable		jolly	
21.		flexible		rigid	
22.		tired		rested	
23.		hesitant		sure	
24.		composed		restless	
25.		without energy		energetic	
26.		useless		useful	
27.		sluggish		animated	
28.		strong		weak	

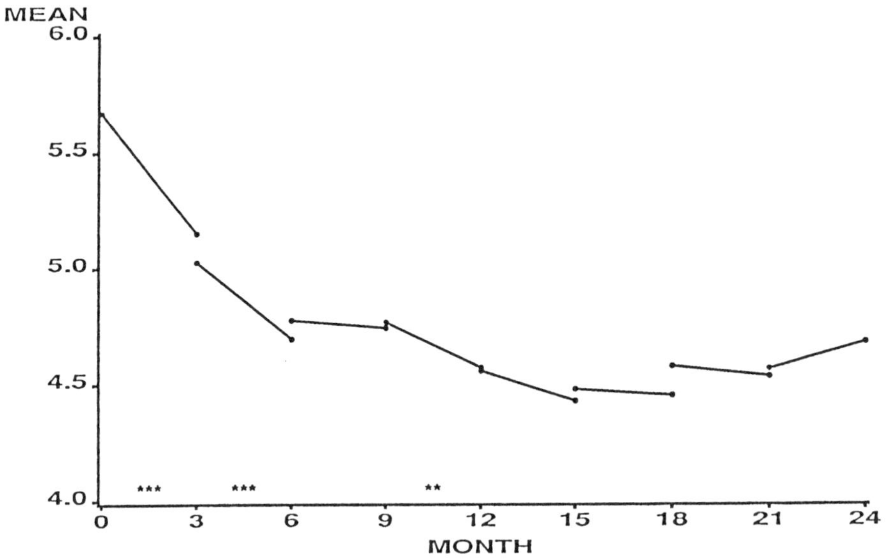

Fig. 6. Preliminary evaluation of mean coping scores from postmenopausal patients (Trials VII and IX) based on the Personal Adjustment to Chronic Illness Scale (PACIS) used in the International Breast Cancer Study Group quality-of-life instrument. Lower scores indicate less effort to cope with the disease (i.e., improved adjustment). In the pairwise analyses shown, the lines connect mean values provided by patients who had both assessments, thus adjusting for patient cohort effects. * $p < .1$, ** $p < .05$, *** $p < .01$

210 patients provide data for the last 2 time points (months 21 and 24).

Significant improvements in adjustment with time from initial diagnosis are observed (Fig. 6). The average score of 32 (square root = 5.67) at diagnosis improves to an average score of 21 (square root = 4.55) within one year of diagnosis. This represents over a 33% improvement in coping score over time.

The coping score is also sensitive to differences in adjustment for the various treatment options. Postmenopausal patients in Trial VII receive either tamoxifen alone (TAM), 3 months of CMF combination chemotherapy plus tamoxifen (TAM + early CT), 3 cycles of late CMF at months 9, 12, and 15 plus tamoxifen (TAM + late CT), or both early and late chemotherapy plus tamoxifen (TAM + early CT + late CT). Scores for patients receiving TAM alone are consistently lower (improved adjustment) than those for patients who receive chemotherapy. At one year from study entry, average coping scores were 16 for TAM, 19 for TAM + early CT, and 25 for TAM + late CT (with or without early CT). Patients in the latter group were receiving a single CMF cycle at the time of the 12-month assessment.

The coping score (PACIS) is a practical, easily administered 1-item scale that is sensitive to global changes over time and to treatment-induced changes in the patients' quality of life.

Can Quality of Life Measures Be Used to Compare Costs and Benefits of Treatment?

In previous issues of the Monograph Series we have described the TWiST and Q-TWiST methods designed to incorporate aspects of quality of life into adjuvant chemotherapy comparisons. Overall survival time for each treatment separately is partitioned into periods with toxic effects of treatment (TOX), those following systemic symptomatic relapse (REL), and those without symptoms and toxicity (TWiST). Quality-adjusted TWiST (Q-TWiST) enables the periods TOX and REL to be multiplied by utility coefficient weights and added to TWiST to form a measure of benefit for each treatment [30,31].

The Q-TWiST method can be retrospectively applied in clinical trials using the databases that are normally available [32]. However, integrating the patients' own value judgments into the analyses was impossible because of the lack of prospectively collected quality-of-life information. The next step in the development of the method is to include patient-derived psychosocial data into the analyses to enable improved assessment of costs and benefits. Patient-derived information can be used in 2 ways: 1) to define more precisely the specific events occurring during the chronic course of the disease which constitute periods of time that can be classified as TOX and REL as distinct from TWiST (longitudinal information), and 2) to provide

utility assessment for defining appropriate values for weighing costs and benefits. This will enable the values associated with different periods of time to better reflect the perceptions of the patients rather than be based exclusively upon statistical assumptions.
The occurrence of late toxicities due to treatment might be used to define an additional amount of time with decreased quality of life denoted by L-TOX (late toxicity). In this way a variety of experiences that influence the patients' quality of life can be integrated into the overall evaluation and comparison of treatment effects, and summarised by an assessment of the amount of time gained for one treatment approach compared with another. Further research in this area to define more clearly the benefits of adjuvant therapy against the costs of available modalities is required to achieve a better understanding for the appropriate use of treatments for patients with operable breast cancer.

Summary

Evaluating adjuvant treatment effects for patients with breast cancer is difficult due to the heterogeneity of the disease, the relatively low event rate (especially for those with node-negative disease), and the modest effects of systemic treatments available today. A long follow-up time is also required in order to demonstrate treatment effects which tend to emerge late, such as those associated with the use of endocrine therapies (e.g., ovarian ablation, or tamoxifen). Within the framework of randomised trials, the proportion of the patient population observed to benefit continually changes over time. Thus, some emphasis on the amount of time gained by the treated patients compared with the controls (both presently and in the future) is required for patient care decision-making.
Some of the ways used to summarise and announce treatment effects often do not accurately reflect the real magnitude of the effects and actual benefits achievable for the patient. Issues include interpretation of: a) the p-value as a measure of treatment effect; b) results from subgroup analysis; c) results from meta-analysis, and d) data concerning the perception of the patients regarding *their* view on well being.
a) The p-value is often incorrectly interpreted as a measure of treatment benefit while in fact it is a measure of the statistical uncertainty of an observed outcome (i.e., a small p-value indicates a low probability that the observed results might be due to chance alone). A p-value greater than 0.05 may reflect too few events (due to too few patients, too low a risk of an event, and/or too short a follow-up interval) rather than no treatment effect. We recommend that, in addition to the p-value, some estimate of the relative reduction in the risk of an event along with its 95% confidence interval be presented.
b) Subgroup analyses are important to define treatment effects within groups with different prognoses, recognising that multiple comparisons increase the chance of a false positive result. Thus, subgroup analyses are facilitated by relying on the estimates of relative treatment effect and by avoiding the use of the p-value to declare incorrectly that, "treatment is effective for one subgroup but not for another."
c) Meta-analysis or overview (the systematic combination of quantitative results from many studies evaluating the same endpoint) is used to increase the number of observed events, and thus increase the chance that a given treatment effect will yield statistically significant observed differences. Risks of meta-analysis include the over-reliance on the no-treatment-interaction assumption when estimating the magnitude of treatment effects, and the over-interpretation of indirect comparisons that are not protected by a randomised design.
d) Clinical trials of adjuvant therapies usually measure the efficacy of treatments by comparing disease-free survival or overall survival. Integration of methods which evaluate life spent with "a given quality" is necessary in order to assist the decision-making process.
Although data are not available as yet, it is likely that the benefit from adjuvant therapies in early breast cancer will be even larger after a long period of follow-up compared to the short-term treatment effects upon which our judgement of benefit is currently based. Integrating quality-of-life-oriented research into the trials, developing alternative methods to describe costs and benefits from adjuvant

systemic therapies, and increasing the public acceptance of clinical research in general and randomised trials in particular will provide a more accurate evaluation of treatments and will reduce the time required to obtain meaningful results.

Acknowledgements

Supported in part by Grant No. CA-06516 from the National Cancer Institute, DHHS and by Grant No. PBR-53 from the American Cancer Society and by generous gifts from the Swiss Cancer League, the Cancer League of Ticino, the Australian Cancer Society, the Swedish Cancer Society, the Frontier Science and Technology Research Foundation, and the Swiss Group for Clinical and Epidemiologic Cancer Research. We thank the patients, nurses, data managers and physicians who participate in the International Breast Cancer Study Group (formerly Ludwig Group), and especially Karen Price, Harriet Petersen and Mary Isley, who assisted in the preparation of the manuscript.

REFERENCES

1 Fisher B, Redmond C, Dimitrov NY, et al: A randomized clinical trial evaluating sequential methotrexate and fluorouracil in the treatment of patients with node-negative breast cancer who have estrogen-receptor-negative tumors. N Engl J Med 1989 (320): 473-478

2 The Ludwig Breast Cancer Study Group: Prolonged disease-free survival after one course of perioperative adjuvant chemotherapy for node-negative breast cancer. N Engl J Med 1989 (320):491-496

3 Henderson IC, Hayes DF, Parker LM, et al: Adjuvant systemic therapy for patients with node-negative tumors. Cancer 1990 (65):2132-2147

4 Kaplan EL, Meier, P: Nonparametric estimation from incomplete observations. J Am Stat Assoc 1958 (53):457-481

5 Peto R: Statistical aspects of cancer trials. In: Halnan KE (ed) Treatment of Cancer. Chapman and Hall, London 1982 pp 867-871

6 Early Breast Cancer Trialists' Collaborative Group: Effects of adjuvant tamoxifen and of cytotoxic therapy on mortality in early breast cancer: an overview of 61 randomized trials among 28,896 women. N Engl J Med 1988 (319):1681-1692

7 Early Breast Cancer Trialists' Collaborative Group (EBCTCG): Treatment of Early Breast Cancer: Worldwide Evidence in 1985-1990. A systematic overview of all available randomized trials in early breast cancer of adjuvant endocrine and cytotoxic therapy. Oxford University Press Monograph, Oxford 1990

8 Goldhirsch A, Gelber RD for the Ludwig Breast Cancer Study Group: Adjuvant chemo-endocrine therapy or endocrine therapy alone for postmenopausal patients: Ludwig studies III and IV. In: Senn HJ, Goldhirsch A, Gelber RD, Osterwalder B (eds) Adjuvant Therapy of Primary Breast Cancer, Recent Results in Cancer Research: Vol 115. Springer Verlag, Berlin 1989 pp 153-162

9 Gelber RD, Goldhirsch A: The concept of an overview of cancer clinical trials with special emphasis on early breast cancer. J Clin Oncol 1986 (4):1696-1703

10 Brunner KW, Sonntag RW, Martz G, et al: Controlled study in the use of combined drug therapy for metastatic breast cancer. Cancer 1975 (36):1208-1219

11 Priestman TJ, Baum M: Evaluation of quality of life in patients receiving treatment for advanced breast cancer. Lancet 1976 (i):899-901

12 Coates AS, Gebski V, Bishop JF, et al for the Australian New Zealand Breast Cancer Trials Group: Improving quality of life during chemotherapy for advanced breast cancer. A comparison of intermittent and continuous treatment strategies. N Engl J Med 1987 (317):1490-1495

13 Maguire P, Selby P, on behalf of the Medical Research Council's Cancer Therapy Committee Working Party on Quality of Life: Assessing quality of life in cancer patients. Br J Cancer 1989 (60):437-440

14 Donovan K, Sanson-Fisher RW, Redman S: Measuring quality of life in cancer patients. J Clin Oncol 1989 (7):959-968

15 Moinpour CM, Feigl P, Metch B, et al: Quality of life end points in cancer clinical trials: review and recommendations. JNCI 1989 (81):485-495

16 Levine MN, Guyatt GH, Gent M, et al: Quality of life in stage II breast cancer: An instrument for clinical trials. J Clin Oncol 1988 (6):1798-1810

17 Gelber RD, Goldhirsch A, Castiglione M, for the International Breast Cancer Study Group: The duration of a life of quality should become the focus of "quality-of-life" studies (letter). J Clin Oncol 1989 (7):542-543

18 Aitken RCB: Measurement of feelings using visual analogue scales. Proc Royal Soc Med 1969 (62):989-996

19 Priestman TJ, Baum M, Jones V, Forbes J: Comparative trial of endocrine versus cytotoxic treatment in advanced breast cancer. Br Med J 1977 (1):1248-1250

20 Coates AS, Fischer Dillenbeck C, McNeil DR, et al: On the receiving end -II. Linear analogue self assessment (LASA) in evaluation of aspects of the quality of life in cancer patients receiving therapy. Eur J Cancer Clin Oncol 1983 (19):1633-1637

21 Coates AS, Glasziou P, McNeil D: On the receiving end-III. Measurement of quality of life during cancer chemotherapy. Ann Oncol 1990 (1):213-317

22 Rahe RH: The pathway between subjects' recent life changes and their near-future illness reports: representative results and methodological issues. In: Dohrenwand BS and Dohrenwand BP (eds) Stressful Life Events: Their Nature and Effects. Wiley and Sons, New York 1974

23 Cassileth BR, Lusk EJ, Miller DS, et al: Psychosocial correlates of survival in advanced malignant disease? N Engl J Med 1985 (312): 1551-1555

24 Kneier AW, Temoshok C: Repressive coping reactions in patients with malignant melanoma as compared to cardiovascular disease patients. J Psychosomatic Res 1984 (28):145-155

25 Gotay CC: Why me? Attributions and adjustment by cancer patients and their mates at two stages in the disease process. Social Sci and Med 1985 (20):825-831

26 Hürny C, Bernhard J, Schatzmann E, Cassileth BR: What does the Personal Adjustment to Chronic Illness Scale (PACIS) measure? In: Holland J, Lesko L, Massie MJ (eds) Current Concepts in Psycho-Oncology and AIDS. Memorial Sloan-Kettering Cancer Center postgraduate course syllabus, Sept 17-19, 1987

27 Rogentine GN, van Kammen DP, Fox BH, et al: Psychological factors in the prognosis of malignant melanoma: a prospective study. Psychosomatic Ned 1979 (41):647-655

28 Zerssen D v: Klinische Selbstrbeurteilungs-Skalen (KSb-S) aus dem Münchener Psychiatrischen Informations-System (PSYCHI München). Die Befindlichkeits-Skala-Parallelformen Bf-S und Bf-S'-Manual. Beltz, Weinheim 1976

29 Zerssen D v: Clinical self-rating (CSRS) of the Munich Psychiatric Information System (PSYCHIS

Munchen). In: Sartorius N, Ban TA (eds) Assessment of Depression. Springer-Verlag, Heidelberg 1986, pp 270-303

30 Goldhirsch A, Gelber RD, Simes RJ, et al. for the Ludwig Breast Cancer Study Group: Costs and benefits of adjuvant therapy in breast cancer: A quality-adjusted survival analysis. J Clin Oncol 1989 (7):36-44

31 Glasziou PP, Simes RJ, Gelber RD: Quality adjusted survival analysis. Stat Med 1990 (9):1259-1276

32 Gelber RD, Goldhirsch A, Cavalli F for the International Breast Cancer Study Group: Quality-of-life-adjusted evaluation of a randomized trial comparing adjuvant therapies for operable breast cancer. Ann Intern Med 1991 (114):621-628

Adjuvant Chemoendocrine Therapies In Pre- and Postmenopausal Breast Cancer
("Can you teach an old dog new tricks ?")

Aron Goldhirsch[1], Monica Castiglione [2] and Richard D. Gelber [3]

1 Division of Oncology, Ospedale San Giovanni, Bellinzona, Ospedale Civico, Lugano, and Ospedale Beata Vergine, Mendrisio, Switzerland
2 Institut für medizinische Onkologie & International Breast Cancer Study Group Operation Office, Bern, Switzerland
3 Harvard Medical School, Harvard School of Public Health, and Dana-Farber Cancer Institute, Boston, MA, U.S.A.

Most breast cancer patients who remain disease free after local and regional treatment eventually relapse and die of or with overt metastases. This is true regardless of whether they received an appropriate local therapy. The current hypothesis ascribes the failure to obtain freedom from disease to occult micrometastatic disease already present at the time of diagnosis and first surgery [1]. This hypothesis has acquired indirect support from the results of clinical trials which showed no additional advantage in terms of disease-free or overall survival for a more radical local therapy [2,3].

There is evidence that occult metastases can still be eliminated by current therapeutic means, but that the patient with overt metastatic disease is incurable. These observations lead in turn to substantially different attitudes towards the treatment of patients in these two distinct clinical situations.

Long before the present hypothesis of disease spread (presence of micrometastases at diagnosis), adjuvant systemic therapy was applied in a form of hormonal ablative treatment consisting of ovarian radiation [4]. At that time, observations made of tumour regression after oophorectomy justified investigations of ablative therapy in patients with operable disease after completion of the local treatment.

Systemic adjuvant chemotherapy was based upon observations of substantial rates of response to cytotoxic agents of measurable metastatic disease. In addition, the first hypothesis concerning their value as adjuvant treatment was related to the attempt to kill cells which detach during operation. The detached cells were at that time considered to be responsible for the subsequent development of overt metastases. This hypothesis of perioperative migration of cells with metastatic potential has been abandoned in favour of one which argues for the presence of micrometastatic disease at the time of primary diagnosis [5].

Experimental observations which have helped to guide the use of adjuvant systemic therapy after surgical removal of the primary tumour have been made on the basis of animal models [6-10]. There is an inverse relationship between the number of viable tumour cells in the animal and response to treatment with cytotoxic agents, i.e., the smaller the number of tumour cells the greater the chemotherapeutic effect. The time of administration also influences the effectiveness of adjuvant systemic therapy. If the surgery has reduced the number of cells to micrometastases consisting of no more than 100 cells, the optimal timing for chemotherapy to potentially eradicate all cells is immediately after operation. In fact, adjuvant therapy after surgery increases the cure rate in animal models in contrast to both delayed administration of drugs and their use without surgical tumour reduction [11]. In an attempt to explain the failure of adjuvant therapy to achieve cure in most of the treated humans despite the fact that a first-order-kinetics drug action might have predicted otherwise, the following issues arise:

i) Tumour heterogeneity as related to the cell cycle, cellular metabolism, and drug availability within a tumour mass.
ii) Resistance to treatment. Among the causes for drug resistance, which may be intrinsic or acquired, are some which are related to the timing of the drug administration. In fact, early administration of cytotoxic drugs, based upon an experimental system, is hypothesised to avert formation of resistant tumour cells [12].
iii) The growth of tumour cells is hypothesised to follow Gompertzian kinetics in which plateaus of slow or no growth are interrupted by random growth spurts [13]. These spurts may be favoured by treatment-free intervals, and represent periods of higher susceptibility to cytotoxics. According to this latter hypothesis the best therapy to avert metastasis is one which follows therapy-free intervals.
Combined chemoendocrine therapy has been postulated as one of the strategies aimed to overcome some of the mechanisms of resistance, specifically, tumour heterogeneity. In fact, endocrine manipulations may act on different subpopulations of malignant cells than those sensitive to the cytostatic or cytolytic action of chemotherapy. Thus, the combined effect of both treatment modalities might result in an additive benefit in terms of cell kill.
Analysing data of trials in advanced disease, all conducted prior to the era of routine oestrogen receptor determination, one may clearly note that the combination of chemotherapy with tamoxifen, diethylstilboestrol, or progestines yielded higher response rates as compared to chemotherapy alone in postmenopausal patients. The overall survival in these series did not seem to favour the synchronous combination of the 2 modalities, especially in the patients with a less aggressive disease presentation [14].
The use of combined chemo- and endocrine therapies in the adjuvant setting is even more controversial. The theoretical argument states that endocrine manipulations may decrease cell turnover, and thus increase resistance to cytotoxic agents of more slowly proliferating micrometastatic breast cancer cells.
Factors involved in interpreting results related to this issue are illustrated by 3 trials. In the National Surgical Adjuvant Breast and Bowel Project (NSABP) Trial B-09, 779 patients were randomised to receive either PF (L-PAM and 5-fluorouracil) or the combination of the 2 cytotoxics with tamoxifen (PFT) [15]. The results showed a qualitative difference of response according to age and steroid hormone receptor status: While patients with ER+ and PR+ primaries in both age groups (i.e., pre- and postmenopausal) benefited from the adjuvant combination in terms of disease-free survival (DFS), there was a tendency for the patients with one of the receptor types classified as negative who received chemoendocrine therapy to have a shorter DFS and overall survival (OS), especially if premenopausal. One explanation for this derives from experiments showing a clear antagonism between tamoxifen and both L-PAM and 5-fluorouracil, in which the endocrine agent inhibits the cytotoxic efficacy of the 2 chemotherapeutic agents [16].
Based upon these experimental data, the results of the NSABP Trial may be interpreted: In younger women, especially those with ER- tumours, for whom the degree of efficacy of chemotherapy is essential for control of disease, a reduced effect of the combination might be due to the antagonism between the cytotoxics and tamoxifen. In contrast, for patient subpopulations which are more responsive to tamoxifen therapy (postmenopausal age, receptor-positive tumours), the effect of the hormone therapy is sufficient to produce some benefit. In favour of this hypothesis one may mention the German (GABG) trial with a direct comparison between the 2 treatments, tamoxifen and multi-agent chemotherapy. A significant advantage in favour of the cytotoxic regimen was observed in the premenopausal cohort, and one for the tamoxifen therapy was observed in the postmenopausal women [17].
Another trial which demonstrated the different role of the combination of chemo- and endocrine therapy in different ages was the trial of the Italian Group (GROCTA). Five hundred and four postmenopausal and premenopausal patients with N+ breast cancer were included [18]. The trial compared endocrine therapy alone with tamoxifen (T) with chemotherapy (CT= CMF regimen) and chemoendocrine treatment (CT+T). The results are displayed in Table 1. The trial accrued exclusively patients with ER+ tumours and, therefore, adds information about the combination of chemoendocrine therapy in

Table 1. Results of the GROCTA trial presented for pre- and postmenopausal and for nodal groups in terms of events of interest (either relapses or deaths) under the form of observed events/expected events (O/E: <1.00 indicated benefit). 504 patients had node-positive, oestrogen receptor-positive (ER+) breast cancer

	Tamoxifen (T) (x 5 yrs)	CMF(CT)	CT+T
Events*			
All patients	0.92	1.55	0.64
Premenopausal	1.14	1.17	0.70
Postmenopausal	0.76	1.98	0.60
N+ 1-3	0.87	1.56	0.72
N+ >3	0.94	1.45	0.63
Deaths			
All patients	0.79	1.55	0.71
Premenopausal	0.92	1.28	0.78
Postmenopausal	0.70	1.85	0.66
N+ 1-3	0.62	1.56	0.92
N+ >3	0.85	1.45	0.66

* Events included all relapses, second malignancies, and death, whichever occurred first

this cohort. The benefit from the combination was mainly evident in patients with a large number of positive nodes, i.e., with a more aggressive presentation.

These results were not confirmed by the 2 ECOG trials in which chemoendocrine therapy has been compared to chemotherapy alone (in postmenopausal patients also to observation alone), and in which no significant difference between the treatment groups could be observed. In fact, in the trial for 551 premenopausal patients (EST 5177) comparing CMF vs CMFP vs CMFPT, all for 12 cycles, the outcomes were similar also for the subgroups defined by ER status and by number of nodes involved. In the trial (EST 6177) for 224 postmenopausal women, comparing CMFPT with CMFP and with observation, the results were practically similar for all treatment groups. Only in the ER-negative subpopulation some advantage was observed for the chemoendocrine therapy. It must be stressed that tamoxifen was used exclusively for the duration of 1 year.

Some evidence exists that prolonging the duration of treatment with tamoxifen beyond cessation of initial chemoendocrine therapy might provide additional benefit, especially if DFS is used as the endpoint. The issue of continuing tamoxifen beyond the chemotherapy was studied in another ECOG trial (4181) in which 962 postmenopausal patients with N+ disease, and with either ER+ or ER- tumours were included. The patients were randomised to one of the following 3 treatment options: CMFPT x 12, then continuation of tamoxifen for 5 years or, CMFPT x 12 then observation or, CMFPT x 4, then observation. Continued tamoxifen seemed to yield the longest DFS [19].

The benefit from the treatment of patients with tamoxifen after cessation of either chemotherapy alone or after combined CMF and tamoxifen still remains to be defined. Similarly, the late effects of ovarian ablation in premenopausal women seem to extend beyond the effects of initial chemotherapy, providing an "endocrine maintenance" treatment. The role of this therapy must also be clarified. Two trials of the International Breast Cancer Study Group (IBCSG: formerly Ludwig Group) have reached 10 years of median follow-up. The presentation of their results might provide additional insights about the late effects of combined chemoendocrine therapy for both premenopausal and postmenopausal women with breast cancer.

IBCSG (Ludwig) Trial II

Premenopausal and perimenopausal women who had histologically-confirmed, non-inflammatory, unilateral breast carcinoma with four or more metastatic lymph nodes in the axilla were included in the trial. Premenopausal and perimenopausal status was defined by at least one of the following criteria: normal menstruation, amenorrhoea for less than 1 year, biochemical evidence of ovarian function, amenorrhoea for 1 to 3 years in patients younger than 52 years old, or hysterectomy without bilateral oophorectomy for patients younger than 56 years old. Surgery was at least a total mastectomy and axillary clearance. Tests to exclude metastatic disease and to verify normal marrow, renal and hepatic functions were prospectively defined and conducted. Follow-up studies were also standardised [20,21].

Between July 1, 1978, and August 31, 1981, 356 patients were randomised to receive either adjuvant chemotherapy (the CMFp combination) or adjuvant surgical oophorectomy followed by the same cytotoxic regimen. This consisted of cyclophosphamide (C) 100 mg/m^2 orally, daily , days 1-14, methotrexate (M) 40 mg/m^2 i.v. and 5-fluorouracil (F) 600 mg/m^2 i.v. both given on days 1 and 8 of the 28-day cycle. Prednisone (p) 7.5 mg per day (5 mg a.m., 2.5 mg p.m.), was given orally, continuously. In both groups the CMFp regimen was given for 12 courses. Adjuvant treatment (chemotherapy or oophorectomy) had to start within 6 weeks of mastectomy. Three hundred and twenty-seven patients (92%) were eligible and evaluable. Causes for exclusion were described in previous reports [21]. The distribution of relevant patient characteristics is given in Table 2.

The participating laboratories adopted standard methods for oestrogen receptor assays of primary tumour. Oestrogen receptor levels of ≥ 10 fmol/mg cytosol protein were considered positive and values below this, negative. Oestrogen receptor results were available in 61% of the patients.

For analysis of disease-free survival, failure was defined as any recurrence, appearance of a second malignant neoplastic disease, or death without evidence of cancer, whichever occurred first. The Kaplan-Meier method [22] was used to estimate survival distributions for disease-free survival, overall survival and types of failure. The 2-sided logrank proce-

Table 2. Patient entry and characteristics for 327 evaluable patients included in Trial II

		TREATMENTS	
	Total	**CMFp**	**Oophorectomy + CMFp**
Total no. randomised	356	176	177
No evaluable patients	327	161	166
(% of total)	(92)	(90)	(94)
Age (%)			
≤ 39 years	27	30	25
≥ 40 years	73	70	75
Nodes involved (%)			
4-6 N+	48	49	46
7-10 N+	24	20	29
>10 N+	28	31	25
Hormone receptor status* (%)			
ER+ (≥ 10)	33	28	37
ER- (0-9)	28	26	31
ER unknown	39	46	32

* Femtomole/mg cytosol protein

dure [23] was used to assess the statistical significance of treatment differences between the survival distributions. Times were measured from the date of randomisation which had to be within 6 weeks from mastectomy. Tests of significance for treatment effects were carried out adjusting for prognostic factors (degree of nodal involvement, tumour size, pathological grade and oestrogen receptor status) using the Cox proportional hazard regression models [24]. Estimates of relative treatment effect expressed as hazard ratios, their 95 percent confidence intervals, and 2-sided p-values were obtained from Cox models including a covariate for treatment.

Results

The disease-free survival (DFS) and the overall survival (OS) percentages at 5 and at 10 years and hazard ratios providing estimates of relative treatment effect are displayed in Table 3. Based on the entire population, a reduction in the risk of both relapse and death was observed for the oophorectomy plus CMFp group that was not statistically significant. Separate analyses of the ER+ cohort yielded treatment-effect estimates that achieve statistical significance of p = .07 and p = .05 for DFS and OS, respectively.
Figures 1 and 2 display the disease-free survival (DFS) and the overall survival (OS) Kaplan-Meier curves for the entire study population by treatment. The outcome by treatment for each of the subpopulations with known oestrogen receptor concentration in the primary tumour (ER+ and ER-) are described in Figure 3 (DFS for ER+ and ER-), and Figure 4 (OS for ER+ and ER-). As previously reported, the advantage in favour of the oophorectomised patients appeared only beyond 4 years follow-up time.
At 120 months median observation time, 235 patients (72%) relapsed, developed a nonbreast malignancy, or died without apparent cancer. Five patients developed non-breast malignancy, 3 in the CMFp group with melanoma, gastric and endometrial cancer (1 each), and 2 in the oophorectomy plus CMFp group with gastric and colon cancer (1 each), 1 patient in the oophorectomy plus CMFp group died of unknown cause without apparent cancer. One hundred and ninety-five patients (60 %) died.
The percentages of patients divided by first site of relapse are displayed in Table 4. Relapses were subdivided into types maintaining an order which reflects a hierarchy of prognostic value. The treatment differences in types of first site of relapse are mainly due to the differences between the percentage of bone involvement: 29% of chemotherapy patients and 23% of the combined chemo-endocrine therapy patients relapsed first in this site.

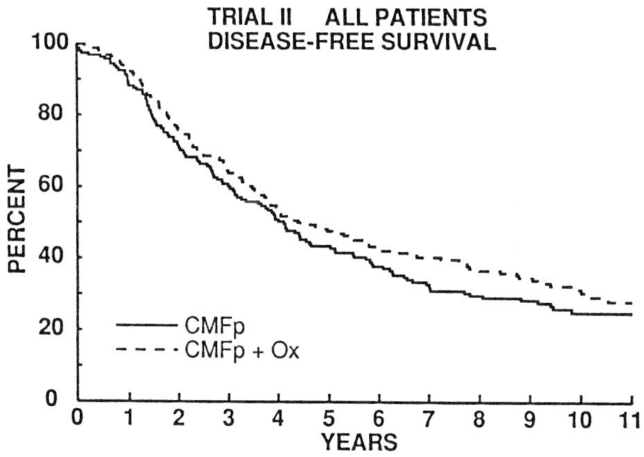

Fig. 1. Disease-free survival for 327 premenopausal and perimenopausal patients with 4 or more positive axillary lymph nodes entered in Trial II at 10 years' median follow-up. See Table 3 for statistical analyses

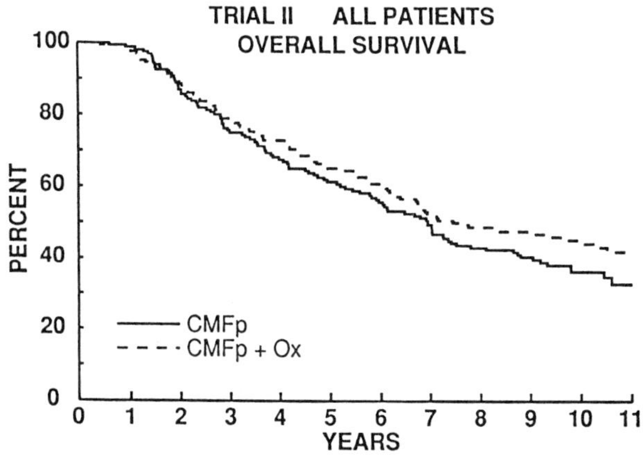

Fig. 2. Overall survival for 327 premenopausal and perimenopausal patients with 4 or more positive axillary lymph nodes entered in Trial II at 10 years' median follow-up. See Table 3 for statistical analyses

Table 3. DFS and OS percentages and hazard ratios* for 327 evaluable premenopausal and perimenopausal patients with N+ in 4 or more lymph nodes included in Trial II at 10 years median' follow up. ER+ are considered those with values of ≥10 fmol / mg cytosol protein

DFS	No. Pts.	DFS % 5-yr	10-yr	Hazard ratio* (95%	confidence interval)	p-value
All patients						
CMFp	161	43	25	.86	(.66-1.10)	0.23
Ox + CMFp	166	48	32			
ER+						
CMFp	45	40	17	.66	(.43-1.03)	0.07
Ox + CMFp	62	55	34			
ER-						
CMFp	42	40	31	1.03	(.64-1.67)	0.90
Ox + CMFp	51	59	23			
ER unknown						
CMFp	74	47	27	.81	(.52-1.25)	0.34
Ox + CMFp	53	47	37			
Age < 40 years						
CMFp	49	43	23	.90	(.55-1.47)	0.67
Ox + CMFp	41	46	29			
Age ≥ 40 years						
CMFp	112	44	25	.84	(.62-1.14)	0.27
Ox + CMFp	125	48	33			

OS	No. Pts.	OS % 5-yr	10-yr	Hazard ratio* (95%	confidence interval)	p-value
All patients						
CMFp	161	61	36	.83	(.63-1.10)	0.19
Ox + CMFp	166	65	44			
ER+						
CMFp	45	64	30	.61	(.37-1.00)	0.05
Ox + CMFp	62	73	52			
ER-						
CMFp	42	50	33	.97	(.60-1.55)	0.89
Ox + CMFp	51	57	30			
ER unknown						
CMFp	74	66	42	.87	(.54-1.41)	0.58
Ox + CMFp	53	64	89			
Age < 40 years						
CMFp	49	58	36	.91	(.54-1.53)	0.72
Ox + CMFp	41	66	40			
Age ≥ 40 years						
CMFp	112	63	36	.81	(.58-1.12)	0.20
Ox + CMFp	125	65	46			

* Hazard ratio for Ox + CMFp relative to CMFp. A value of 1.0 indicates no treatment difference; values less than 1.0 indicate a lower risk of relapse or death for Ox + CMFp compared with CMFp. Hazard ratios, 95% confidence intervals, and 2-sided p-values were calculated using Cox models with treatment as a single covariate

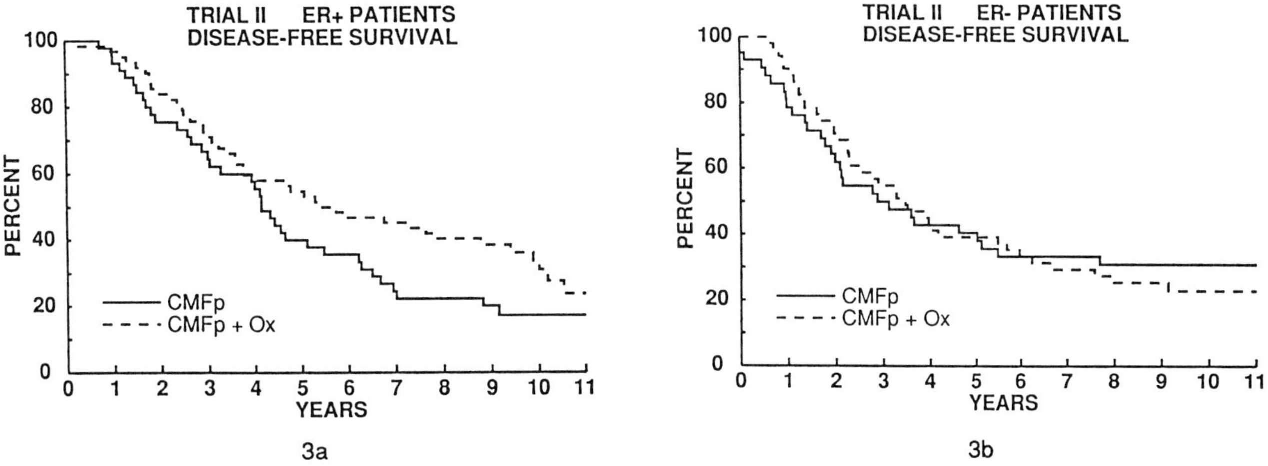

Fig. 3. Disease-free survival for 107 patients with ER+ tumours (3a) and 93 patients with ER- tumours (3b) entered in Trial II at 10 years' median follow-up. See Table 3 for statistical analyses

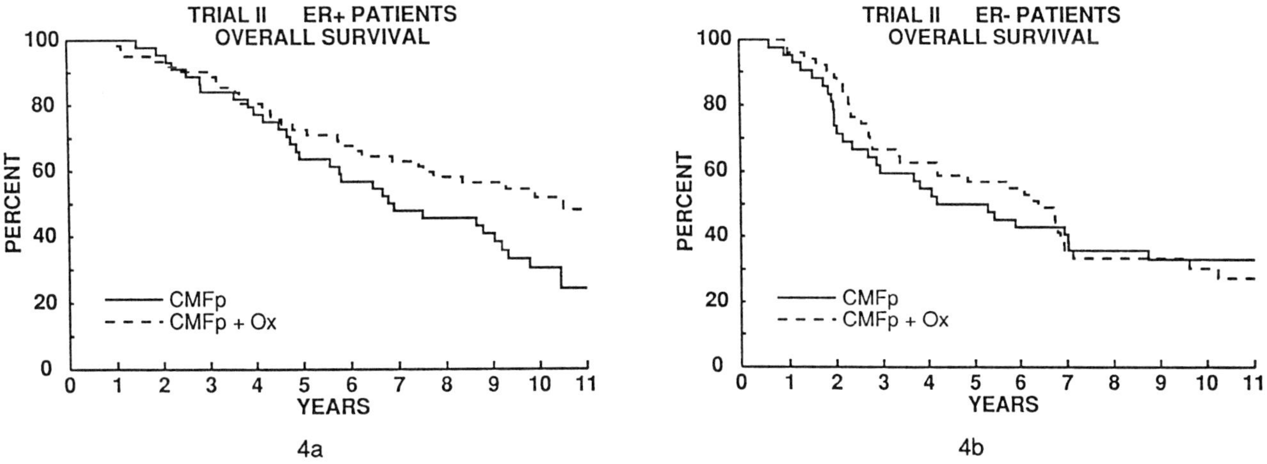

Fig. 4. Overall survival for 107 patients with ER+ tumours (4a) and 93 patients with ER- tumours (4b) entered in Trial II at 10 years' median follow-up. See Table 3 for statistical analyses

Only one study had a similar design to the IBCSG Trial II, i.e., chemotherapy *versus* chemotherapy preceded by surgical oophorectomy. This recently reported South West Oncology Group (SWOG) trial accrued 314 patients with N+ and ER+ primaries from October 1979 to July 1989 [25]. The low patient entry obtained during a 10-year accrual period may be at least partially attributed to the chemotherapy regimen: weekly (continuous) CMFVP for the duration of one year. At a median follow-up of about 5 years the outcome of the 2 treatment groups differed very little, far from showing any statistically significant advantage. These early results from the SWOG trial confirmed the initial observation made from IBCSG Trial II, which had shown no significant effects of oophorectomy, if added to chemotherapy, within the first few years of follow-up [20]. The updated 8-year results from Trial II at 96 months' median follow-up have been published [26]. At that time DFS and OS differences in the ER+ cohort did not reach statistical significance, although a modified logrank analysis for the follow-up period beyond 4 years yielded a significant difference. The additional follow-up currently reported confirms the continued late benefit for the oophorectomy group, especially for

Table 4. Sites of first relapse or death without overt breast cancer: percentages of patients relapsing at a given site out of the patients in each treatment group in Trial II at 10 years' median follow-up

	CMFp (%)	Oophorectomy + CMFp (%)
Scar	10	10
Contralateral breast	1	2
Regional ± local	11	10
Distant metastases	50	46
Soft tissue	4	4
Bone	29	23
Viscera	17	19
Second primary (not breast)	2	1
Death without relapse	0	1
Total failed	74 (120 / 161)	69 (115 / 166)

patients with ER+ primaries. The recently published 30-year results of the Norwegian ovarian radiation trial clearly illustrated in the 169 premenopausal patients included in the study that the treatment benefit in terms of both DFS and OS continues to increase during follow-up [27].
We hypothesise that the use of ablative hormone therapy with or without another endocrine manipulation may be a way to improve upon results of adjuvant cytotoxic therapies in premenopausal women with average risk operable breast cancer.

IBCSG (Ludwig) Trial III

Postmenopausal women 65 years old or younger who had histologically-confirmed, non-inflammatory, unilateral breast carcinoma with at least one metastatic lymph node in the axilla were included in the trial. Postmenopausal status was defined by at least one of the following criteria: amenorrhoea for 1 year or more if the women was 52 years old or older; amenorrhoea for 3 years or more in patients younger than 52 years old, biochemical evidence of ceased ovarian function. Also patients who had undergone hysterectomy without bilateral oophorectomy had to be at least 56 years old in order to be considered postmenopausal. Surgery was at least a total mastectomy and axillary clearance. All other aspects of eligibility, definitions of patient characteristics and logistics of conduct of the trial, including follow-up, were similar to Trial II.
Between July 1, 1978, and August 31, 1981, 503 patients were randomised to receive either no adjuvant treatment (Observation), endocrine therapy alone with tamoxifen 20 mg/day and prednisone 7.5 mg/day (5 mg a.m., 2.5 mg p.m.) for the duration of 12 months (p+T), or the combination of chemotherapy and endocrine therapy (the CMFp+T combination) which consisted of cyclophosphamide (C) 100 mg/m^2 orally, daily, days 1-14, methotrexate (M) 40 mg/m^2 i.v. and 5-fluorouracil (F) 600 mg/m^2 i.v. both given on days 1 and 8 of the 28-day cycle. Prednisone (p) and tamoxifen (T) were given orally, continuously as above. The CMFp+T regimen was given for 12 courses.
Four hundred and sixty-three patients (92%) were eligible and evaluable. Causes for exclusion were described in previous reports [21], and the distribution of relevant patient characteristics is given in Table 5. The evaluation of data was conducted using the same methods as described above for Trial II.

Results

The disease-free survival and the overall survival percentages at 5 and at 10 years are displayed in the first part of Table 6. Hazard ratios and 95 percent confidence intervals showing relative treatment effects between each pair of treatments are given in the second part of Table 6. Results for all patients

Table 5. Patient entry and characteristics for 463 evaluable patients included in Trial III

	Total	TREATMENTS Observ.	p+T	CMFp+T
Total no. randomised	503	168	164	171
No. evaluable patients	463	156	153	154
(% of total)	(92)	(93)	(93)	(90)
Age				
Median	59	59	59	60
Range	40-65	40-65	45-65	46-65
Nodes involved (%)				
1-3	56	55	54	58
≥4	44	45	46	42
Hormone receptor status* (%)				
ER+ (≥10)	33	34	29	38
ER - (0-9)	18	21	20	12
ER unknown	49	45	51	50

* Femtomole/mg cytosol protein

Table 6. DFS and OS percentages and hazard ratios** for 463 evaluable postmenopausal patients with N+ breast cancer included in Trial III at 10 years' median follow-up. ER+ are considered those with values of ≥10 fmol/mg cytosol protein. P-values refer to the test of heterogeneity. Statistically significant differences between p+T and CMFp+T in a pairwise comparison (p ≤ 0.05) are indicated with an asterisk

	No. pts.	DFS % 5-yr	10-yr	p-value	OS % 5-yr	10-yr	p-value
All patients							
Observ.	156	30	18	<0.0001	58	35	0.08
p+T	153	42	29*		63	41	
CMFp+T	154	58	38*		70	49	
ER+							
Obser.	53	30	20	0.02	72	40	0.80
p+T	45	55	32		80	41	
CMFp+T	58	60	30		74	48	
ER-							
Obser.	33	30	21	0.02	45	33	0.17
p+T	30	20	17*		37	23	
CMFp+T	19	63	47*		63	49	
ER unknown							
Obser.	70	30	15	<0.0001	56	32	0.18
p+T	78	44	31*		63	47	
CMFp+T	77	57	42*		70	50	

Table 6. (contd.)

	Pairwise hazard ratios** (95% confidence intervals)			
	DFS		OS	
All patients				
p+T: Observ.	.74	(.57-0.95)	.93	(.70-1.23)
CMFp+T: Observ.	.50	(.38-0.65)	.71	(.53-0.96)
CMFp+T: p+T	.69	(.52-0.91)	.78	(.57-1.06)
ER+				
p+T: Observ.	.61	(.38-0.98)	.96	(.56-1.62)
CMFp+T: Observ.	.57	(.37-0.88)	.84	(.51-1.40)
CMFp+T: p+T	.95	(.59-1.53)	.88	(.52-1.51)
ER-				
p+T: Observ.	1.22	(.70-2.11)	1.34	(.75-2.41)
CMFp+T: Observ.	.45	(.22-0.94)	.66	(.30-1.44)
CMFp+T: p+T	.38	(.18-0.79)	.50	(.23-1.08)
ER unknown				
p+T: Observ.	.67	(.46-0.96)	.78	(.51-1.18)
CMFp+T: Observ.	.45	(.30-0.67)	.67	(.44-1.02)
CMFp+T: p+T	.67	(.45-0.99)	.88	(.57-1.36)

** Hazard ratios and 95% confidence intervals were calculated using Cox models with treatment as a single covariate. Confidence intervals that do not include the null hypothesis value of 1.0 indicate pairwise comparisons that are significant at the $p \leq .05$ level (not adjusted for multiple comparisons)

and for subpopulations defined by oestrogen receptor content of the primary (ER+, ER-, ER unknown) are shown. One year of endocrine therapy (p+T) reduced the risk of relapse and death compared with observation for all subpopulations except the ER- cohort. Differences in DFS were statistically significant ($p \leq .05$) while those for overall survival were not. The CMFp+T chemoendocrine therapy regimen reduced the risk of relapse and death for all subpopulations compared with either observation or p+T alone. With re-

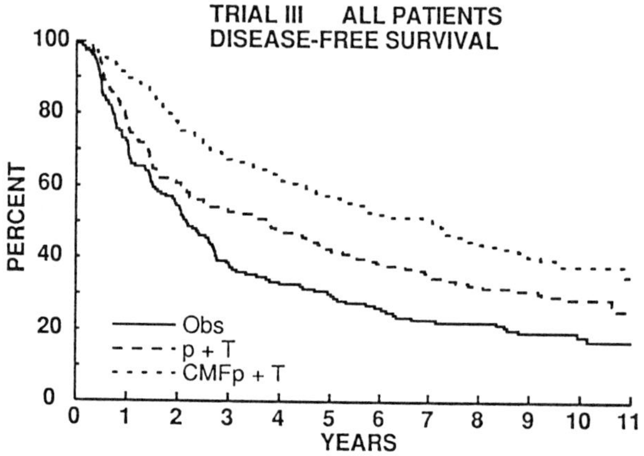

Fig. 5. Disease-free survival for 463 postmenopausal patients with positive axillary lymph nodes entered in Trial III at 10 years' median follow-up. See Table 6 for statistical analyses

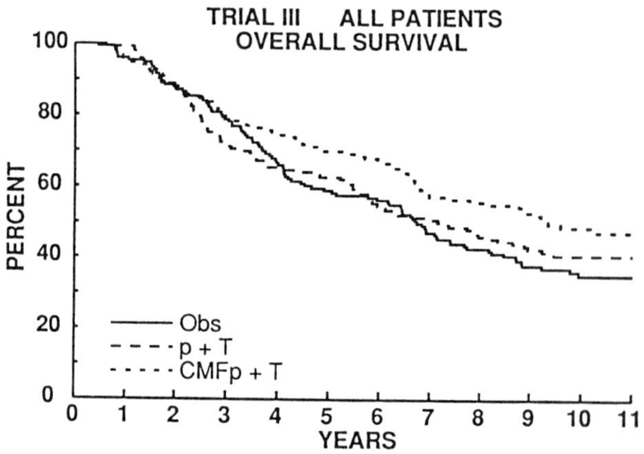

Fig. 6. Overall survival for 463 postmenopausal patients with positive axillary lymph nodes entered in Trial III at 10 years' median follow-up. See Table 6 for statistical analyses

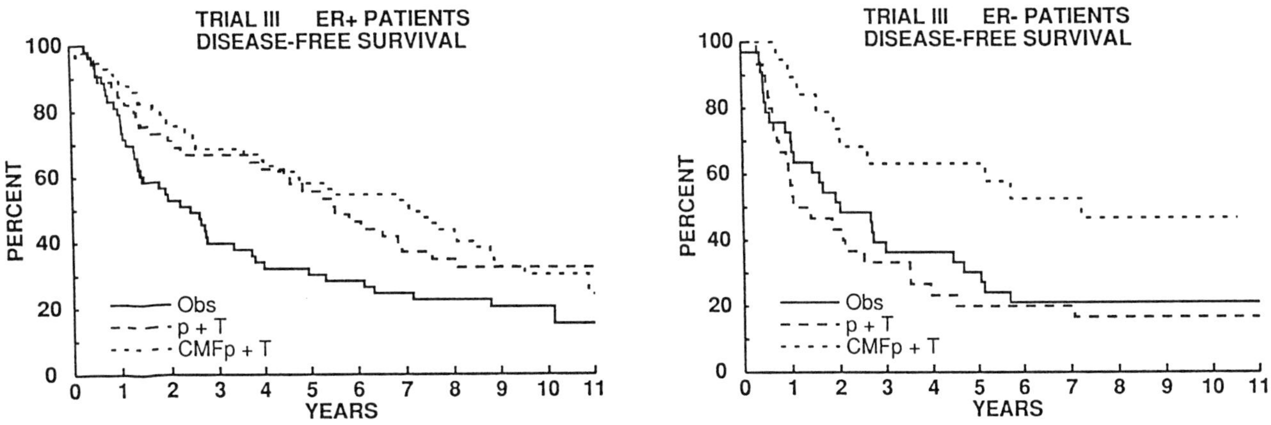

7a 7b

Fig. 7. Disease-free survival for 156 patients with ER+ tumours (7a) and 82 patients with ER- tumours (7b) entered in Trial III at 10 years' median follow-up. See Table 6 for statistical analyses

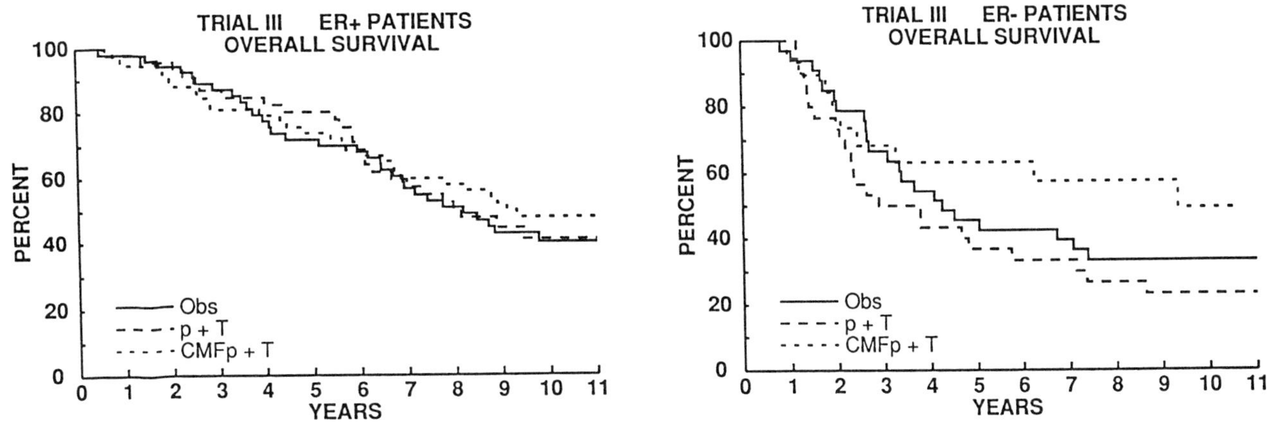

8a 8b

Fig. 8. Overall survival for 156 patients with ER+ tumours (8a) and 82 patients with ER- tumours (8b) entered in Trial III at 10 years' median follow-up. See Table 6 for statistical analyses

spect to DFS, all pairwise comparisons were statistically significant in favour of CMFp+T, except for CMFp+T versus p+T for the ER+ cohort. For OS among all patients, CMFp+T reduced mortality compared with both observation (p = .03) and p+T (p = .11). Adding cytotoxic chemotherapy to endocrine therapy improves outcome, especially for patients with ER- primaries.

Figures 5 and 6 display the disease-free survival (DFS) and the overall survival (OS) Kaplan-Meier curves for the entire study population by treatment. The outcomes by treatment for each of the subpopulations with known oestrogen receptor concentration in the primary tumour (ER+ and ER-) are described in Figure 7 (DFS for ER+ and ER-) and Figure 8 (OS for ER+ and ER-).

At 120 months median observation time, 332 patients (72%) relapsed or developed a non-breast malignancy or died without apparent cancer. Fifteen patients developed a non-breast second cancer, 5 in each treatment group. These were as follows: Observation: endometrium (2), gall bladder (2), colorectal (1); p+T: cervical-vagina, gastric, gall bladder, rectal, and acute myelocytic leukemia (AML) (one each); CMFp+T: pancreatic, oesophageal, renal cell, bladder, and AML (one each). Nineteen patients died without apparent cancer, 2 in the observation group, 5 in p+T, and 12 in CMFp+T. These were as follows: Observation: asthma and myocardial infarction (1 each); p+T: cardio- or cerebrovascular (4 patients, 1 within the first year), liver cirrhosis (1); CMFp+T: cardio- or cerebrovascular (7 patients, 3 within the first year), sepsis in a diabetic subject (1), peritonitis due to perforated ulcer (1 patient, within the first year), bleeding from a duodenal ulcer (1), unknown cause (2). Two hundred and sixty-six patients (57.5 %) died.

The percentages of patients divided by first site of relapse are displayed in Table 7. Relapses were subdivided into types maintaining an order which reflects a hierarchy of

Table 7. Sites of first relapse or death without overt breast cancer: percentages of patients relapsing at a given site out of the patients in each treatment group in Trial III at 10 years' median follow-up

	Observ.		p+T		CMFp+T	
Scar	17		12		6	
Contralateral breast	4		1		1	
Regional ± local	17		9		8	
Distant metastases	39		44		35	
Soft tissue		1		1		1
Bone		16		21		16
Viscera		22		22		18
Second primary (not breast)	3		3		3	
Death without relapse	1		3		8	
Total failed	81 (127 / 156)		72 (111 / 153)		61 (94 / 154)	

Table 8. Sites of first relapse or death without overt breast cancer by ER status of the primary tumour: percentages of patients relapsing at a given site out of the patients in each treatment group in Trial III at 10 years' median follow-up

	Observ.	p+T	CMFp+T
ER+ Tumours			
Scar	26	7	9
Contralateral breast	6	2	2
Regional ± local	13	4	10
Distant metastases	30	45	38
Second primary (not breast)	4	4	3
Death without relapse	2	4	7
Total Failed	81 (43 / 53)	67 (30 / 45)	69 (40 / 58)
ER- Tumours			
Scar	9	20	5
Contralateral breast	3	0	0
Regional ± local	18	13	0
Distant metastases	49	50	37
Second primary (not breast)	0	0	5
Death without relapse	0	0	5
Total failed	79 (26 / 33)	83 (25 / 30)	53 (10 / 19)

prognostic value. The treatment differences in types of first site of relapse were mainly due to the differences between the percentage of local and regional relapses. Only the combined chemoendocrine therapy (CMFp+T) group experienced a reduction in first relapses in distant sites, compared with the 2 other treatment groups. A more detailed analysis indicated that these differences could be attributed mainly to visceral metastases (± others). The analysis of patterns of first relapse in the subpopulations with known ER status in the primary tumours is shown in Table 8. While in patients with ER+ tumours adjuvant therapy reduced first relapses in sites which are associated with a better subsequent prognosis (i.e., local and regional recurrences, as well as contralateral breast disease), in patients with ER- tumours the effect upon first relapse seemed to be confined to distant disease.

Discussion

A large amount of data will be provided by the update of the Worldwide Overview of all randomised trials investigating adjuvant systemic therapy. In fact, the first edition of this work was less informative for combined chemoendocrine therapies because only few trials were available in which the combination was studied [28]. While the Overview update will allow the overall estimation of the magnitude of treatment effects for the combination, the most interesting aspects of chemoendocrine therapy will be still provided by individual trials because they relate to the way the 2 modalities are combined. The following questions seem relevant for evaluation in current and future trials:

- Continuous administration of tamoxifen beyond the initial chemotherapy.
- Concomitant or sequential use of chemotherapy and endocrine therapy.
- Delayed use of tamoxifen in premenopausal women who become postmenopausal after adjuvant chemotherapy.
- Effects of chemoendocrine therapy by ER status.
- Effects of endocrine treatment-free intervals upon susceptibility to reintroduction of delayed chemotherapy.
- Effects of adjuvant combination endocrine therapies, administered either sequentially or concomitantly, and combined with chemotherapy.

Studying these issues represents attempts to improve the use of combined chemo- and endocrine therapy. It is likely, however, as demonstrated in the premenopausal patients, that the effects of the endocrine component of the combination will become evident only late during follow-up, a fact which led us [20] and others [25] to mistakenly declare the ineffectiveness of the combination relying upon early evaluations. A meta-analysis might, however, be the only method to identify early differences among treatment groups, despite the fact that trials in which the above issues are investigated are not easily comparable.

Increasing the variety of questions asked in trials requires an increase in patient accrual. It is important, therefore, that efforts be carried out to make clinical research acceptable in a way that no one will find it in conflict with The Physician's Oath of the World Medical Association: "Concern for the interests of the subject must always prevail over the **interests** of science and society" [29]. Specifically, judging the issue of adjuvant therapies in terms of **interests** of the individual patient, one encounters difficulties in the definition of benefit. In fact, for the evaluation of therapies for operable breast cancer, due to the heterogeneity of the disease and to the time frame in which results and benefits emerge, there are very few alternatives to randomised trials to define patient benefit from a given treatment. These include the study of sequential series in the case which allows a fast evaluation of an endpoint of interest (e.g., response of the primary tumour to a given treatment) [30]. It is, therefore, unfortunate that randomised clinical trials are being defined *globally* as an unethical and non-human methodology [31]. Neither breast conserving procedures, nor adjuvant systemic therapies would have been recognised as valuable treatments for women with breast cancer without the convincing evidence of a randomised study. It is also due to insufficient acceptance of such clinical research that information about the effects of endocrine and chemotherapies in the adjuvant setting is still missing for both premenopausal and postmenopausal breast cancer patients. We have limited data to assume that some forms of combination between adjuvant chemotherapy and endocrine therapies yield a larger benefit than each modality given alone.

Summary

Adjuvant systemic therapy has been shown to reduce relapses in treated women and to prolong their survival. Despite a significant benefit for treated patients, the proportion of those who relapse despite treatment is still very large. Combined chemo- and endocrine therapies show some increasing advantage compared to each modality given alone as adjuvant treatment. The 10-year results of 2 International (Ludwig) Breast Cancer Group Trials (II and III) which studied this combined approach are presented showing the advantage obtainable with the combinations. Furthermore, ways to improve upon study designs to investigate available endocrine and chemotherapies for premenopausal and postmenopausal patients are discussed.

Acknowledgements

We thank the patients, nurses, data managers, and physicians who participate in the International Breast Cancer Study Group (formerly Ludwig Group). We also acknowledge the support of the Ludwig Institute for Cancer Research which initiated the trials, and the support of the Frontier Science and Technology Research Foundation, the Swiss Cancer League, the Cancer League of Ticino, the Swedish Cancer Society, the Australian Cancer Society, the Australia-New Zealand Breast Cancer Study Group, and the Swiss Group for Clinical and Epidemiological Cancer Research which enabled the continuation of the trials.

REFERENCES

1 Henderson IC, Canellos GP: Cancer of the breast: the past decade. N Engl J Med 1980 (302): 17-30, 78-90
2 Veronesi U, Cascinelli N, Greco M et al: Prognosis of breast cancer patients after mastectomy and dissection of internal mammary nodes. Ann Surg 1985 (202): 702-707
3 Fisher B, Redmond C, Poisson R et al: Eight-year results of a randomized clinical trial comparing total mastectomy and lumpectomy with or without irradiation in the treatment of breast cancer. N Engl J Med 1989 (320): 822-828
4 Cole MP: Prophylactic compared with therapeutic x-ray artificial menopause. 2nd Tenovus Workshop of Breast Cancer, 1970 pp 2-11
5 Berlin NI: Research strategy in cancer: screening, diagnosis, prognosis. Hosp Practice 1975 (10): 83-91
6 Martin DS, Fugman RA: A role of chemotherapy as an adjunct to surgery. Cancer Res 1957 (17):1098-1101
7 Martin DS: Clinical implications of the interrelationship of tumor size and chemotherapeutic response. Ann Surg 1960 (151): 97-100
8 Martin DS, Hayworth PE, Fugman RA: Enhanced cures of spontaneous murine mammary tumors with surgery, combination chemotherapy, and immunotherapy. Cancer Res 1970 (30): 709-716
9 Karrer K, Humphreys SR: Continuous and limited courses of cyclophosphamide (NSC 26271) in mice with pulmonary metastases after surgery. Cancer Chemother Rep 1967 (51): 439-449
10 Mayo JG, Laster WR, Andrews CM, Schable FM: Success and failure in the treatment of solid tumors. III. Cure of metastatic Lewis lung carcinoma with methyl-CCNU (NSC 94551) and surgery-chemotherapy. Cancer Chemother Rep 1972 (56): 183-195
11 Martin DS, Fugman RA, Stolfi RL, et al: Solid tumor animal model therapeutically predictive for human breast cancer. Cancer Chemother Rep 1975 (59): 89-109
12 Goldie JH, Coldman AJ: A mathematic model for relating the drug sensitivity of tumors to spontaneous mutation rate. Cancer Treat Rep 1979 (63): 1727-1733
13 Retsky MW, Wardwell RH, Swartzendruber DE, et al: Prospective computerized simulation of breast cancer: comparison of computer predictions with nine sets of biological and clinical data. Cancer Res 1987 (47): 4982-4997
14 Cavalli F, Pedrazzini A, Martz G, Jungi WF, Brunner KW, Goldhirsch A, Mermillod B, Alberto P: Randomized trial of 3 different regimens of combination chemotherapy in patients receiving simultaneously a hormonal treatment for advanced breast cancer. Eur J Cancer Clin Oncol 1983 (19): 1615-1624
15 Fisher B, Redmond C, Brown A, et al: Adjuvant chemotherapy with and without tamoxifen: five-year results from the National Surgical Adjuvant Breast

and Bowel Project Trial. J Clin Oncol 1986 (4):459-471

16 Osborne CK: Effects of estrogens and antiestrogens on cell proliferation. Implications for treatment of breast cancer. In: Osborne CK (ed) Endocrine Therapies in Breast and Prostatic Cancer. Kluwer Academic Publishers, Boston, 1988 pp111-129

17 Kaufmann M, Jonat W, Caffier H, et al: Adjuvant systemic risk adapted cytotoxic +/- tamoxifen therapy in women with node-positive breast cancer. In: Salmon SE (ed) Adjuvant Therapy Of Cancer V. Grune & Stratton, Orlando, 1987 pp 337-346

18 Boccardo F, Rubagotti A, Bruzzi P, et al : Chemotherapy versus tamoxifen versus chemotherapy plus tamoxifen in node-positive, estrogen receptor-positive breast cancer patients: Results of a multicentric Italian study. J Clin Oncol 1990 (8):1310-1320

19 Falkson HC, Gray R, Wolberg WH, Falkson G: Adjuvant therapy of postmenopausal women with breast cancer- An ECOG phase III study. Proc ASCO 1989 (8):19

20 Ludwig Breast Cancer Study Group: Chemotherapy with or without oophorectomy in high-risk premenopausal patients with operable breast cancer. J Clin Oncol 1985 (3):1059-1067

21 Goldhirsch A, Gelber RD for the Ludwig Breast Cancer Study Group. Adjuvant treatment for early breast cancer: The Ludwig Breast Cancer Studies. NCI Monogr 1986 (1): 55-70

22 Kaplan EL, Meier P: Nonparametric estimation from incomplete observation. J Am Statist Assoc 1958 (53): 457-481

23 Peto R, Pike MC, Armitage P, et al: Design and analysis of randomized clinical trials requiring prolonged observation of each patient. Br J Cancer 1977 (35): 1-39

24 Cox DR: Regression models and life tables (with discussion). J R Stat Soc B (Methodology). 1972 (34): 187-220

25 Rivkin S, Green S, Metch B, et al: Adjuvant chemotherapy (CMFVP) vs oophorectomy followed by chemotherapy (OCMFVP) for premenopausal women with ER+ operable breast cancer with positive (+) axillary lymph nodes: An Intergroup study. Proc ASCO 1991 (10): 47

26 The International Breast Cancer Study Group: Late effects of adjuvant oophorectomy and chemotherapy upon pre-menopausal breast cancer patients. Ann Oncol 1990 (1):30-35

27 Nissen-Meyer R: Primary breast cancer: The effect of primary ovarian irradiation. Ann Oncol 1991 (2): 343-346

28 Early Breast Cancer Trialists' Collaborative Group.Effects of adjuvant tamoxifen and of cytotoxic therapy on mortality in early breast Cancer: An overview of 61 randomized trials among 28,896 women. N Engl J Med 1988 (319): 1681-1692

29 Report on Medical Ethics. World Med Assoc Bull 1949 (1):109-111

30 Bonadonna G, Veronesi U, Brambilla C, et al: Primary chemotherapy to avoid mastectomy in tumors with diameters of three centimeters or more. JNCI 1990 (82): 1537-1545

31 Hellman S, Hellman DS: Of mice but not men. Problems of the randomized clinical trial. N Engl J Med 1991 (324):1585-1589